W9-AUR-103

············ THE ············

KETO
FOR TWO

COOKBOOK

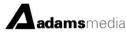

Adams Media
An Imprint of Simon & Schuster, Inc.
57 Littlefield Street
Avon, Massachusetts 02322

Copyright © 2019 by Simon & Schuster, Inc.

All rights reserved, including the right to reproduce this book or portions thereof in any form whatsoever. For information address Adams Media Subsidiary Rights Department, 1230 Avenue of the Americas, New York, NY 10020.

First Adams Media trade paperback edition December 2019

ADAMS MEDIA and colophon are trademarks of Simon & Schuster.

For information about special discounts for bulk purchases, please contact Simon & Schuster Special Sales at 1-866-506-1949 or business@simonandschuster.com.

The Simon & Schuster Speakers Bureau can bring authors to your live event. For more information or to book an event contact the Simon & Schuster Speakers Bureau at 1-866-248-3049 or visit our website at www.simonspeakers.com.

Interior design by Sylvia McArdle
Interior photographs by Audrey Roberts; page 10 © 123RF

Manufactured in the United States of America

10 9 8 7 6 5 4 3 2 1

Library of Congress Cataloging-in-Publication Data
Names: Boyers, Lindsay, author.
Title: The keto for two cookbook / Lindsay Boyers, CHNC.
Description: Avon, Massachusetts: Adams Media, 2019.
Includes index.
Identifiers: LCCN 2019030612 | ISBN 9781507212448 (pb) | ISBN 9781507212455 (ebook)
Subjects: LCSH: Ketogenic diet. | Reducing diets. | Low-carbohydrate diet. | Cooking for two. | LCGFT: Cookbooks.
Classification: LCC RM237.73 .B6933 2019 | DDC 641.5/6383--dc23
LC record available at https://lccn.loc.gov/2019030612

ISBN 978-1-5072-1244-8
ISBN 978-1-5072-1245-5 (ebook)

Many of the designations used by manufacturers and sellers to distinguish their products are claimed as trademarks. Where those designations appear in this book and Simon & Schuster, Inc., was aware of a trademark claim, the designations have been printed with initial capital letters.

The information in this book should not be used for diagnosing or treating any health problem. Not all diet and exercise plans suit everyone. You should always consult a trained medical professional before starting a diet, taking any form of medication, or embarking on any fitness or weight training program. The author and publisher disclaim any liability arising directly or indirectly from the use of this book.

Always follow safety and commonsense cooking protocols while using kitchen utensils, operating ovens and stoves, and handling uncooked food. If children are assisting in the preparation of any recipe, they should always be supervised by an adult.

Contains material adapted from the following title published by Adams Media, an Imprint of Simon & Schuster, Inc.: The Everything® Ketogenic Diet Cookbook by Lindsay Boyers, CHNC, copyright © 2017, ISBN 978-1-5072-0626-3.

LINDSAY BOYERS, CHNC

THE

KETO
FOR TWO
COOKBOOK

100 Delicious, Keto-Friendly Recipes
JUST FOR TWO!

Adams Media
New York   London   Toronto   Sydney   New Delhi

CONTENTS

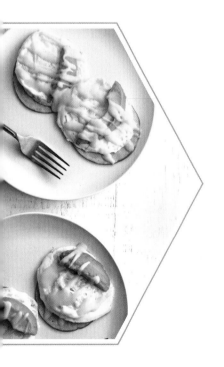

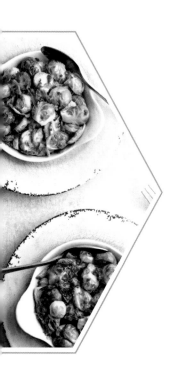

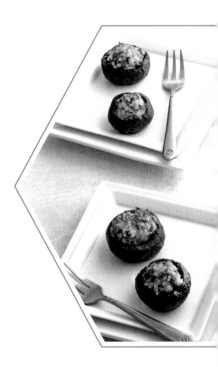

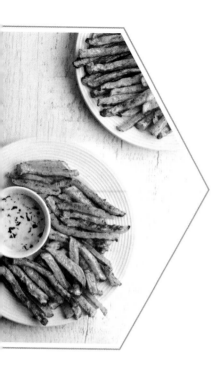

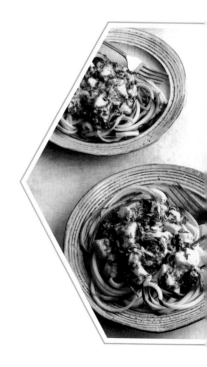

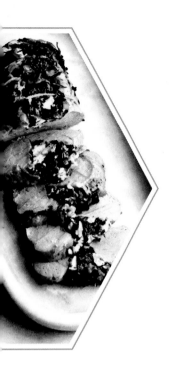

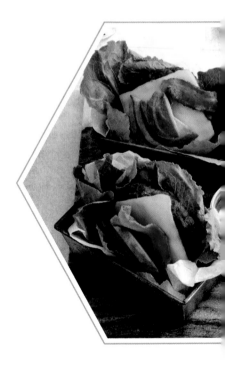

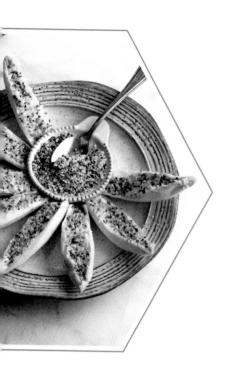

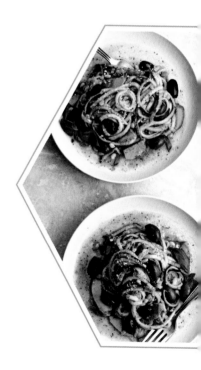

CHAPTER 11

DESSERTS ... 155

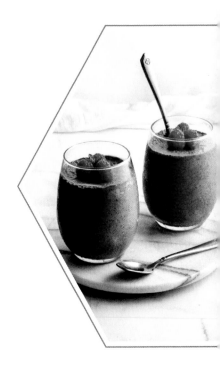

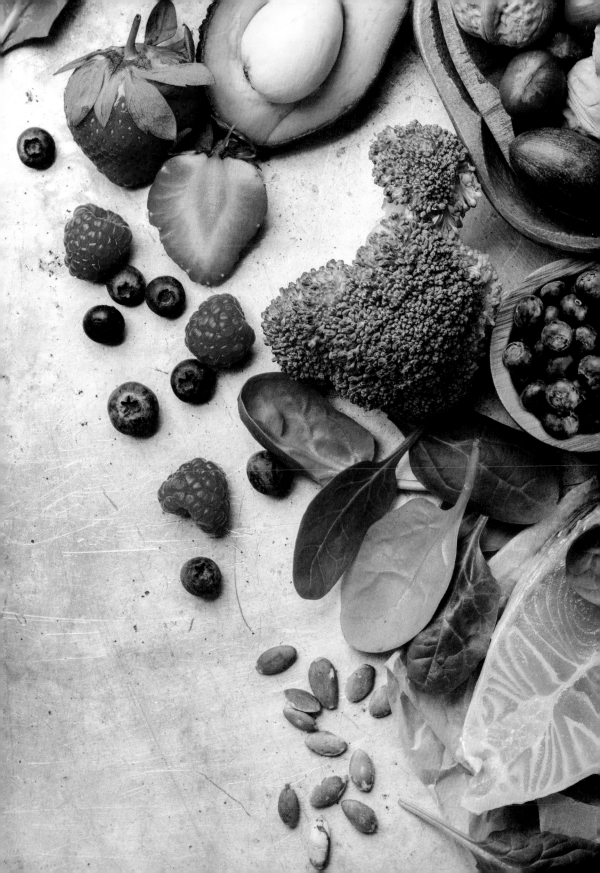

INTRODUCTION

When you're following a keto diet, you need exciting new recipes that can fight the food monotony that often develops. Unfortunately, most keto recipes you'll find are designed to make six servings (or sometimes even more). But when you're only cooking for one or two people, that can translate to *a lot* of leftovers and unused food. Not to mention, wasting precious keto-approved ingredients is definitely not something that you want to do! But now you can eat what you want without wasting food with *The Keto for Two Cookbook*.

Inside, you'll find one hundred delicious keto-approved recipes that cover everything from breakfasts and dinners to snacks and even desserts. There are meals that are designed for meat eaters and others that are vegetarian friendly. You'll also find suggestions on how to easily adapt the recipes to fit your dietary preferences and your taste buds. And the best part? Every recipe in this book is already designed and perfectly portioned for two.

But it's not just the serving size that makes these recipes stand out; they're also already macronutrient-balanced to fit in with your keto lifestyle. Need to know how many net carbs are in each recipe? That information is already listed for you. Trying to boost your fat intake? You'll know exactly how many grams are in each serving so you can make educated choices when designing your meal plan.

The recipes also use ingredients that you probably already have stocked in your pantry or refrigerator. There's nothing unusual or hard to find here. Just simple low-carbohydrate meals that are easy to whip up, but satisfying and delicious enough for even the most sophisticated palates.

Sharing a meal with someone is one of the most basic pleasures in life. With *The Keto for Two Cookbook*, you can spend less time calculating your macros and converting recipes and more time eating while enjoying each other's company.

CHAPTER 1

THE KETOGENIC LIFESTYLE

Lots of things in life are better with a partner—and keto is one of those things. It doesn't matter what it is; any lifestyle change is just easier to stick to when you have support from someone—whether it's your mom, a friend, a romantic partner, or a roommate—and this book was designed with that in mind.

Every recipe in it is perfectly balanced for two, so you can have an easy, satisfying meal without any of the waste that comes from recipes designed for a bigger crowd. Of course, if you want to make more, you can double recipes and use the leftovers for meal prep. But before jumping into the recipes, let's start with a little background for those of you who are new to a ketogenic lifestyle.

HOW YOUR BODY OBTAINS ENERGY

Energy cannot be created. It can only be converted from one form to another. Because of this, your body needs to get energy from somewhere. It uses the food, and the macronutrients from the food, that you eat. The biochemical process of obtaining energy is a complicated one, but it's important to understand the basics so you can get a feel for how the ketogenic diet and ketosis work on a cellular level.

ENERGY FROM CARBOHYDRATES

Although your body is adept at using any food that's available for energy, it always turns to carbohydrates first. When you eat carbohydrates, they are ultimately broken down or converted into glucose, which is absorbed through the walls of the small intestine. From the small intestine, glucose enters into your bloodstream, which naturally causes your blood glucose levels to rise. As soon as the glucose enters your blood, your pancreas sends out insulin to pick it up and carry it to your cells so they can use it as energy.

Once your cells have used all the glucose they need at that time, much of the remaining glucose is converted into glycogen (the storage form of glucose), which is then stored in the liver and muscles. The liver has a limited ability to store glycogen, though; it can only store enough glycogen to provide you with energy for about twenty-four hours. All the extra glucose that can't be stored is converted into triglycerides, the storage form of fat, and stored in your fat cells.

When you don't eat for a few hours and your blood sugar starts to drop, your body will call on the glycogen stored in the liver and muscles for energy before anything else. The pancreas releases a hormone called glucagon, which triggers the release of glucose from the glycogen stored in your liver to help raise your blood sugar levels. This process is called glycogenolysis. The glycogen stored in your liver is used exclusively to increase your blood glucose levels, while the glycogen stored in your muscles is used strictly as fuel for your muscles. When you eat carbohydrates again, your body uses the glucose it gets

from them to replenish those glycogen stores. If you regularly eat carbohydrates, your body never has a problem getting access to glucose for energy and the stored fat stays where it is—in your fat cells.

ENERGY FROM PROTEIN

Protein is the body's least favorite macronutrient to use as energy. This is because protein serves so many other functions in the body. Protein provides structural support to every cell in your body and helps maintain your body tissues. Proteins act as enzymes that play a role in all of the chemical reactions in your body. Without these enzymes, these chemical reactions would be so slow that your body wouldn't be able to carry out basic processes like digestion and metabolism and you wouldn't be able to survive. Proteins also help maintain fluid and acid-base balance, help transport substances such as oxygen through the body and waste out of the body, and act as antibodies to keep your immune system strong and help fight off illness.

Proteins are made up of amino acids. When you eat proteins, your body breaks them down into their individual amino acids, which are then converted into sugars through a process called gluconeogenesis. Your body can use these protein-turned-sugars as a form of energy, but that means your body isn't using the amino acids for those other important functions. It's best to avoid forcing the body to use protein for energy, and you do that by providing it with the other nutrients it needs.

ENERGY FROM FAT

In the absence of carbohydrates, your body turns to fat for energy. The fat from the food you eat is broken down into molecules called fatty acids, which enter the bloodstream through the walls of the small intestine. Most of your cells can directly use fatty acids for energy, but some specialized cells, such as the cells in your brain and your muscles, can't run on fatty acids as they are. To appease these cells and give them the energy they need, your body uses fatty acids to make ketones.

WHAT IS KETOSIS?

In order to convert fat into useable energy, the liver breaks it down into fatty acids and then breaks down these fatty acids into energy-rich substances called ketones or ketone bodies. The presence of ketone bodies in the blood is called ketosis. The goal of a ketogenic diet is to kick your body into long-term ketosis, essentially turning it into a fat-burning machine.

THE CREATION OF KETONES

When following a ketogenic diet, fat is taken to the liver where it is broken down into glycerol and fatty acids through a process called beta-oxidation. The fatty-acid molecules are further broken down through a process called ketogenesis, and a specific ketone body called acetoacetate is formed.

Over time, as your body becomes adapted to using ketones as fuel, your muscles convert acetoacetate into beta-hydroxybutyrate, or BHB, which is the preferred ketogenic source of energy for your brain, and acetone, most of which is expelled from the body as waste.

The glycerol created during beta-oxidation goes through a process called gluconeogenesis. During gluconeogenesis, the body converts glycerol into glucose that your body can use for energy. Your body can also convert excess protein into glucose. Your body does need some glucose to function, but it doesn't need carbohydrates to get it because it does a good job of converting whatever it can into the simple sugar.

KETOSIS AND WEIGHT LOSS

Now that you understand how your body creates energy and how ketones are formed, you may be left wondering how this translates into weight loss. When you eat a lot of carbohydrates, your body happily burns them for energy and stores any excess as glycogen in your liver

or as triglycerides in your fat cells. When you take carbohydrates out of the equation, your body depletes its glycogen stores in the liver and muscles and then turns to fat for energy. Your body obtains energy from the fat in the food you eat, but it also uses the triglycerides, or fats, stored in your fat cells. When your body starts burning stored fat, your fat cells shrink and you begin to lose weight and become leaner.

HOW TO INDUCE KETOSIS

The first step in inducing ketosis is to severely limit carbohydrate consumption, but that's not enough. You must limit your protein consumption as well. Traditional low-carbohydrate diets don't induce ketosis because they allow a high intake of protein. Because your body is able to convert excess protein into glucose, your body never switches over to burning fat as fuel. You can induce ketosis by following a high-fat diet that allows moderate amounts of protein and only a small amount of carbohydrates—or what is called a ketogenic diet.

The exact percentage of each macronutrient you need to kick your body into ketosis may vary from person to person, but in general the macronutrient ratio falls into the following ranges:

- 60–75 percent of calories from fat
- 15–30 percent of calories from protein
- 5–10 percent of calories from carbohydrates

Once you're in ketosis, you have to continue with the high-fat, low-carbohydrate, moderate-protein plan. Eating too many carbohydrates or too much protein can kick you out of ketosis at any time by providing your body with enough glucose to stop using fat as fuel.

SIGNS THAT YOU ARE IN KETOSIS

Signs that you're in ketosis may start appearing after only one week of following a true ketogenic diet, but for some people it can take longer—as much as three months. When signs do start to show, they are pretty similar across the board. Signs of ketosis typically include:

- Bad breath
- Decreased appetite and nausea
- Cold hands and feet
- Increased urinary frequency

- Difficulty sleeping
- Metallic taste in the mouth
- Dry mouth
- Increased thirst

And eventually:

- Increased energy
- Improved mental focus and clarity

"KETO FLU"

"Keto flu," or "low-carb flu," commonly affects people in the first few days of starting a ketogenic diet. Of course, the ketogenic diet doesn't actually cause the flu, but the phenomenon is given the term because its symptoms closely resemble those of the flu. It would be more accurate to refer to this stage as a carbohydrate withdrawal, because that's really what it is. When you take carbohydrates away, it causes altered hormonal states and electrolyte imbalances that are responsible for the associated symptoms. The basic symptoms include headaches, nausea, upset stomach, sleepiness, fatigue, abdominal cramps, diarrhea, and lack of mental clarity, or what is commonly referred to as "brain fog."

The duration of symptoms varies—it depends on you as an individual, but typically a "keto flu" lasts anywhere from a couple of days to a week. In rare cases it can last up to two weeks. Some of the symptoms of the "keto flu" are associated with dehydration, because in the beginning stages of ketosis you lose a lot of water weight, and with that lost fluid you also lose electrolytes. You can replenish these electrolytes by drinking enhanced waters (but make sure they are not sweetened) and drinking lots of homemade bone broth. This may help lessen the severity of the symptoms.

Although these signs are common among many people who follow a ketogenic diet, your experience may be different. Every body is unique, so it's impossible to say exactly what your personal experience will be. Keep in mind that in the early stages of ketosis your symptoms may be unpleasant, but as your body adapts you will begin to experience the benefits of following a ketogenic diet plan.

FAT IS ESSENTIAL TO GOOD HEALTH

If you're still on the fence about consuming so much fat, it's important to remember that fat is an integral part of every cell in your body. This macronutrient is a major component of your cell membranes, which hold each cell together. Every single cell in your body, from the cells in your brain to the cells in your heart to the cells in your lungs, is dependent on fat for survival. Fat is especially important for your brain, which is made up of 60 percent fat and cholesterol.

Fat and cholesterol are used as building blocks for many hormones, which help regulate metabolism, control growth and development, and maintain bone and muscle mass, among many other things. Fat is vital for proper immune function, helps regulate body temperature, and serves as a source of protection for your major organs, surrounding all of your vital organs to provide a sort of cushion for protection against falls and trauma. It also helps boost metabolic function and plays a role in keeping you lean.

Fat is classified as an essential nutrient, which means that you need to ingest it through the foods you eat because the body cannot make what it needs on its own. Fat is composed of individual molecules called fatty acids. Two of these fatty acids, omega-3 fatty acids and omega-6 fatty acids, are absolutely essential for good health. Omega-3 fatty acids play a crucial role in brain function and growth and development, while omega-6 fatty acids help regulate metabolism and maintain bone health. Fat also allows you to absorb and digest other essential nutrients, such as vitamins A, D, E, and K and beta-carotene. Without enough fat in your diet, you wouldn't be able to absorb any of these nutrients and you would eventually develop nutritional deficiencies.

Fat is also a major source of energy for your body. Because each gram contains nine calories, fat is a compact source of energy that your body can use easily and efficiently. Unlike with carbohydrates, which your body can only store in limited amounts, your body has an unlimited ability to store fat for later use. When food intake falls short, such as between meals or while you're sleeping, your body calls on its

fat reservoirs for energy. This physiological process is what the entire ketogenic diet is based upon.

FAT IS NOT THE ENEMY

Fat is not your enemy; sugar is. And that applies to all forms of sugar, not only the granulated stuff that you put in your coffee in the morning. Sure, the sugar in fruit is packaged with vitamin C, potassium, fiber, and other valuable nutrients, which makes it a far superior choice over white sugar, but overdoing it can actually hinder weight loss efforts and set you up for other health problems, particularly if you have blood sugar issues.

EATING FAT DOES NOT MAKE YOU FAT

On the surface, the theory that eating fat makes you fat seems like a no-brainer. Of the three macronutrients—protein, carbohydrates, and fat—fat contains the most calories per gram. Protein and carbohydrates have four calories per gram, while fat contains nine calories per gram. It would make sense that if you cut out fat or replace fat with protein or carbohydrates at each meal, you would be saving yourself calories throughout the course of the day, and while technically this is true, it doesn't lead to sustainable weight loss.

In order to understand why fat doesn't make you fat, you have to understand how you gain weight in the first place. Here's a simple explanation: You start thinking about food and your body secretes insulin in response. The insulin triggers your body to store fatty acids instead of using them for energy, so you get hungry. When you get hungry, you eat. If you're on a low-fat diet, your lunch may consist of two slices of whole-wheat toast with a couple of slices of turkey—no cheese, no mayonnaise—and an apple on the side. If you've subscribed to the low-fat diet theory, this looks like a healthy meal, but in reality it's loaded with carbohydrates that pass through your digestive system quickly, causing significant spikes in blood sugar.

Your body quickly breaks down your high-carbohydrate meal, which sends a rush of glucose into your bloodstream. Your body responds to this glucose by secreting more insulin, which carries the glucose out of your blood and into your cells. Once the glucose levels

drop, you get hungry again, your body secretes more insulin, and the cycle starts over.

Now here's where you'll want to pay close attention. Your body's main regulator of fat metabolism is insulin. Insulin controls lipoprotein lipase, or LPL, an enzyme that pulls fat into your cells. The higher your insulin levels, the more fat LPL pulls into your cells. Translation: When insulin levels increase, you store fat. When insulin levels drop, you burn fat for energy. The main thing that affects insulin levels is carbohydrates, not fat. So when you eat a lot of carbohydrates, your insulin levels increase, which increases your LPL levels, which increases your storage of fat. The goal is to avoid surges and crashes in glucose and insulin and to keep your levels consistent and steady throughout the day. When you do this, your body is better able to handle both glucose and insulin over the long term.

It's important to remember that overdoing it on any of the nutrients will lead to weight gain. Regularly exceeding your caloric needs will cause weight gain regardless of whether you do it with carbohydrates, protein, or fat—but fat is not, and never has been, the major culprit.

DESIGNING YOUR KETOGENIC DIET PLAN

The first thing you need to do to design your ketogenic diet is figure out how many calories you need each day. From there you'll be able to calculate your macronutrient ratio—or the best breakdown of fat, protein, and carbohydrates for you. There are several online calculators that can calculate this number for you, but to do it yourself, you can use a method called the Mifflin-St. Jeor formula, which looks like this:

▸ **Men:** 10 × weight (kg) + 6.25 × height (cm) − 5 × age (y) + 5
▸ **Women:** 10 × weight (kg) + 6.25 × height (cm) − 5 × age (y) − 161

To make this explanation easier, let's try using the equation with a thirty-year-old, 160-pound (72.7 kg) woman who is 5 feet 5 inches (165.1 cm) tall. When you plug this woman's statistics into the Mifflin-St. Jeor formula, you can see that she should be eating 1,448 calories

per day. Now you'll use the estimated macronutrient percentages to calculate how much of each nutrient she needs to consume in order to follow a successful ketogenic diet plan.

CARBOHYDRATES

On a ketogenic diet, carbohydrates should provide only 5–10 percent of the calories you consume. Many ketogenic dieters stay at the low end of 5 percent, but the exact amount you need depends on your body. Unfortunately, there is no one-size-fits-all approach to this, so you'll have to do a little trial and error. You can pick a percentage that feels right for you and try that out for a couple of weeks. If you don't see the results you want, you'll have to adjust your nutrient ratios and calculate them again. Getting 7 percent of your calories from carbohydrates is a good place to start.

To convert this percentage into grams, multiply 7 percent by the total number of calories, which, in the earlier example, is 1,448, and then divide by 4 (since carbohydrates contain 4 calories per gram). The number you're left with—25 in this example—is the amount of carbohydrates in grams you should eat per day.

FAT

Next up is fat. Again, the exact amount you'll need depends on you as an individual, but consuming 75 percent of your calories from fat is a good place to start. To figure out the amount of fat you need in grams, multiply the amount of calories you need (in this example, 1,448) by 75 percent and then divide by 9 (since fat contains 9 calories per gram). The number you're left with is the total grams of fat you need for the day. In this example it's 121 grams.

PROTEIN

Once you've calculated carbohydrates and fat, protein is easy. The remainder of your calories, which equates 18 percent, should come from protein. To figure out this number in grams, multiply the total number of calories by 18 percent and then divide by 4 (since protein contains 4 calories per gram). The number you're left with is the total grams of protein you need for the day. In this example it's 65 grams.

FOODS TO EAT AND AVOID

When following a ketogenic diet, some foods are strictly off-limits, while others fall into a sort of gray area. Regardless of whether foods are "allowed," you still have to make sure that you're staying within your macronutrient ratios. Just because a food is technically allowed doesn't mean you can eat as much of it as you want. Use these recommendations as a guideline, but always make sure that you're staying within your calculated macronutrient ratios.

FATS AND OILS

Fats and oils provide the basis of your ketogenic diet, so you'll want to make sure you're eating plenty of them. The ketogenic diet is not just a fat free-for-all, though. While following a ketogenic diet, there are certain fats that are better for you than others, although which ones fall into which category may surprise you. On the ketogenic diet you should eat plenty of saturated fats in the form of meat, poultry, eggs, butter, and coconut; monounsaturated fats such as olive oil, nuts, nut butters, and avocado; and natural polyunsaturated fats such as tuna, salmon, and mackerel. Avoid highly processed polyunsaturated fats such as canola oil, vegetable oil, and soybean oil. Homemade mayonnaise is also an easy way to add a dose of fat to every meal.

PROTEINS

Many of the fat sources mentioned previously—meat, poultry, eggs, butter, nuts, nut butters, and fish—are also loaded with protein and should be your main protein sources when following a ketogenic diet. Bacon and sausage are other sources of protein that also provide a significant dose of fat, so keep that in mind when including them in your ketogenic diet. When eating protein make sure to stay within your recommended grams for the day, since your body turns excess protein into glucose, which can kick you out of ketosis.

FRUITS AND VEGETABLES

On a ketogenic diet most fruits fall onto the "do not eat" list because even though the sugars are natural, they still raise your blood glucose levels significantly and can kick you out of ketosis. There's not a hard rule—that fruit isn't allowed on a ketogenic diet—but you do need to limit your intake. When you do eat fruit, choose fruits that are high in fiber and lower in carbohydrates, such as berries, and limit your portions.

Vegetables are extremely important on a ketogenic diet. They provide the vitamins and minerals that you need to stay healthy and help fill you up without contributing a lot of calories to your day. You do have to be choosy about which vegetables you eat, though, since some are loaded with carbohydrates. As a general rule, choose dark green or leafy green vegetables, such as spinach, broccoli, cucumbers, green beans, lettuce, and asparagus. Cauliflower and mushrooms are also good choices for a ketogenic diet. Avoid starchy vegetables like white potatoes, sweet potatoes, yams, and corn.

DAIRY

Full-fat dairy products are a staple on the ketogenic diet. You can use butter, heavy cream, sour cream, cream cheese, hard cheese, and cottage cheese to help meet your fat needs. Avoid low-fat dairy products and flavored dairy products, such as fruit yogurt, which is full of sugar; serving for serving, some versions contain as much sugar and carbohydrates as soda. It's especially important to pay attention to quality when choosing dairy products. Dairy from grass-fed cows and raw cheeses are best.

BEVERAGES

As with any diet plan, when it comes to beverages, water is the ideal choice. Make sure to drink at least half your body weight in ounces. Coffee and tea are also permitted on a ketogenic diet, but they must be unsweetened or sweetened with an approved sweetener, such as stevia or erythritol. Avoid sodas, flavored waters, sweetened teas, sweetened lemonade, and fruit juices. You can infuse plain water with fresh herbs, such as mint or basil, to give yourself a little variety.

Avoid grains and sugars in all of their forms on the ketogenic diet. Grains include wheat, barley, rice, rye, sorghum, and anything made from these products. That means no breads, no pasta, no crackers, and no rice. Sugar, and anything that contains sugar, is also not allowed on a ketogenic diet. This includes white sugar, brown sugar, honey, maple syrup, corn syrup, and brown rice syrup. There are many names for sugar on ingredient lists; it's extremely beneficial to familiarize yourself with these names so you'll know when a product contains sugar in any form.

WHEN THE KETOGENIC DIET SHOULD NOT BE USED

While the ketogenic diet is safe for most individuals, there are some people who should not follow the diet plan. If you have certain metabolic conditions or health conditions, talk to your doctor before starting a ketogenic diet.

If you're pregnant or trying to become pregnant, a ketogenic diet may not be right for you. A woman is the most fertile when her body feels satisfied and well nourished. Because ketosis is essentially a starvation state, it's a gamble for women attempting to become pregnant to try this diet. A high level of ketones in the blood may also pose a risk to a developing fetus. While traditional low-carbohydrate diets are okay during pregnancy, you should not limit your carbohydrates to the point of ketosis if you're pregnant.

Achieving success on a ketogenic diet may take some trial and error and a little bit of practice (and patience), but once you get into the routine and reach a state of optimal ketosis your body will adjust accordingly. If you experience any uncomfortable symptoms or hit any roadblocks, contact a functional medicine doctor or a functional nutritionist who can help you troubleshoot and overcome any hurdles.

CHAPTER 2

BREAKFASTS

They say breakfast is the most important meal of the day, but sometimes, especially when you only have a few minutes to get out the door, it's tempting to skip it altogether. While this may work for you if you're combining intermittent fasting with your keto diet plan, if you're not, skipping breakfast can make it more difficult to stick to your plan the rest of the day.

The recipes in this chapter were designed with simplicity in mind. Of course, they're low in carbs, but they also don't require a lot of extra effort, so you can whip up a healthy breakfast for two in no time. In this chapter, you'll find Individual Crustless Quiche, Peanut Butter Pancakes, and even Cinnamon Roll Bars. Whether you're on team savory or team sweet when it comes to breakfast, there's something to make you happy in this chapter.

PEANUT BUTTER PANCAKES

SERVES 2

If you don't eat peanut butter or you want to lower the carb count of these Peanut Butter Pancakes even more, swap out the peanut butter in this recipe for macadamia nut butter instead, which contains 20 grams of fat, but only 2 grams of net carbs per tablespoon serving.

2 ounces cream cheese, softened

2 large eggs

3 tablespoons unsalted, unsweetened peanut butter

¼ teaspoon vanilla extract

⅛ teaspoon ground cinnamon

2 teaspoons coconut oil

PER SERVING
Calories: 431
Fat: 38g
Protein: 14g
Sodium: 176mg
Fiber: 2g
Carbohydrates: 7g
Net Carbohydrates: 5g
Sugar: 3g

1 In a medium mixing bowl, beat cream cheese, eggs, and peanut butter together. Stir in vanilla and cinnamon until mixture is smooth.

2 Melt coconut oil in a large skillet and pour one quarter of peanut butter mixture into the hot pan. Cook 3–4 minutes and then flip. Cook another 2–3 minutes on the second side. Repeat until all batter is cooked.

IS PEANUT BUTTER KETO?

Many people wonder if peanut butter is okay for a keto diet and it is, if you do it right. A 2 tablespoon serving of no-sugar-added peanut butter provides 16 grams of fat and 4 grams of net carbs, which can fit into your keto macros. You just have to make sure you're choosing a peanut butter that doesn't have any added sweeteners or artificial ingredients and sticking to the right portions.

CINNAMON ROLL BARS

SERVES 2

The sugar dragon can come on strong, especially when you're on keto. Although it's best to resist the temptation of your sugar cravings as much as possible, sometimes you just need a sweet, cinnamon-y breakfast for two.

½ cup creamed coconut, cut into chunks

¾ teaspoon ground cinnamon, divided

1 tablespoon coconut oil

1 tablespoon almond butter

PER SERVING

Calories: 269
Fat: 26g
Protein: 3g
Sodium: 8mg
Fiber: 5g
Carbohydrates: 9g
Net Carbohydrates: 4g
Sugar: 2g

1 Line two (6-ounce) quiche dishes with parchment paper.

2 In a small bowl, mix creamed coconut and ¼ teaspoon cinnamon with hands thoroughly. Divide into two equal-sized portions and press into bottom of prepared quiche dishes.

3 In a separate small bowl, whisk coconut oil, almond butter, and remaining ½ teaspoon cinnamon until combined and spread over creamed coconut layer.

4 Place pan in freezer 10 minutes to set.

5 Cut into two equal-sized bars and eat immediately.

HEALTH BENEFITS OF CINNAMON

Some studies show that cinnamon may help improve insulin resistance by balancing blood sugar levels and the way insulin responds to them. To add to that, it's filled with antioxidants, and is anti-inflammatory in nature, so it's an excellent addition to any diet, not just a keto one. Cinnamon is also known to curb hunger, lower blood pressure, and reduce the risk of heart disease.

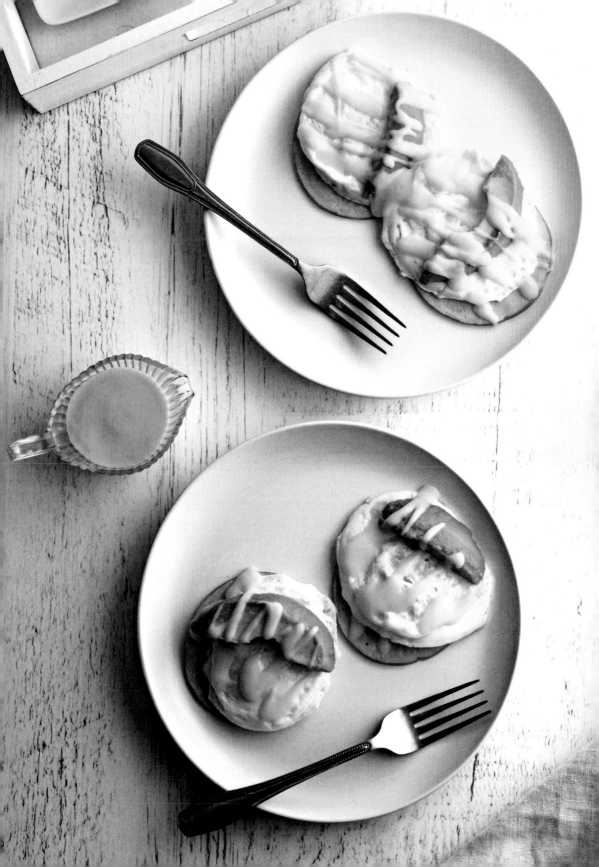

EGGS BENEDICT

SERVES 2

If you're looking for a breakfast for two that feels fancy, but doesn't take a lot of time to prepare, check out this keto-approved Eggs Benedict. Like the traditional version, this one calls for Canadian bacon, but you can use no-sugar-added bacon, no-sugar-added sausage, or prosciutto in its place if you prefer.

4 large egg yolks

½ teaspoon salt

1 tablespoon fresh lemon juice

½ cup plus 1 tablespoon grass-fed butter, divided

4 large whole eggs

4 slices no-sugar-added Canadian bacon, cooked

½ large avocado, peeled, pitted, and cut into 4 slices

PER SERVING

Calories: 845
Fat: 77g
Protein: 26g
Sodium: 1,180mg
Fiber: 2g
Carbohydrates: 6g
Net Carbohydrates: 4g
Sugar: 1g

1 Start by making the hollandaise sauce. Put egg yolks, salt, and lemon juice in a blender and blend until smooth.

2 Put ½ cup butter in a microwave-safe dish and microwave on high until melted and hot, about 45–60 seconds.

3 With egg yolk mixture in blender, turn blender on low speed and slowly pour in the melted butter. The sauce will thicken.

4 Heat a medium skillet over medium-high heat and add remaining 1 tablespoon of butter. Crack whole eggs into pan. Cook 2 minutes and then flip eggs, using care not to break yolks. Cook another 2 minutes or until white is completely cooked, but yolk is still runny.

5 Place Canadian bacon on a plate and top each slice with one egg and one slice avocado. Pour the sauce mixture onto each egg, evenly dividing it among all the eggs.

THE BENEFITS OF GRASS-FED BUTTER

Any type of butter will work in these recipes; however, there is a benefit to going grass-fed. Grass-fed butter contains approximately five times more conjugated linoleic acid, or CLA, which has been shown to help you lose more fat and better maintain your weight loss than butter that comes from conventional cows. It's also higher in omega-3 fatty acids and important vitamins and minerals, like vitamin K.

COCONUT YOGURT

SERVES 2

A lot of commercial yogurts are full of sugar and artificial ingredients that don't just kick you out of ketosis; they almost completely negate any health benefits you'd get from them. Fortunately, it's easy to make your own yogurt at home with only two ingredients that are easy to find.

1 (13.5-ounce) can full-fat coconut milk

1 probiotic capsule

PER SERVING

Calories: 376
Fat: 38g
Protein: 4g
Sodium: 24mg
Fiber: 0g
Carbohydrates: 5g
Net Carbohydrates: 5g
Sugar: 0g

1 Pour coconut milk into a blender. Open probiotic capsule and dump contents into blender. Blend until smooth.

2 Pour mixture into two separate sealable oven-safe containers. Seal containers and place on a baking sheet.

3 Put baking sheet with containers in the oven and turn oven light on. Keep the oven door closed and leave containers in the oven 24 hours.

4 Store in the refrigerator up to seven days.

PICKING A PROBIOTIC

There are so many probiotics available that it can be difficult to know which one to pick. Choose a probiotic that contains at least seven different strains of bacteria and at least five billion organisms per dose. Make sure to store the probiotic per the manufacturer's instructions, as exposure to high heat and too much light can kill the bacteria, rending the probiotic useless. Take a quick look at the ingredient list too. Some probiotics can have sugar hiding out there.

INDIVIDUAL CRUSTLESS QUICHE

SERVES 2

These Individual Crustless Quiches are the perfect option for a Sunday sit-down breakfast. They're easy to put together and come out of the oven in 15 minutes, so you can spend less time in the kitchen and more time enjoying your breakfast partner's company.

4 large eggs

¼ cup heavy cream

1 tablespoon olive oil

3 tablespoons chopped mushrooms

¼ cup fresh spinach

2 tablespoons minced white onion

¼ cup chopped broccoli

¼ teaspoon black pepper

¼ teaspoon salt

¼ teaspoon garlic powder

¼ cup shredded Cheddar cheese

¼ cup shredded Colby jack cheese

PER SERVING

Calories: 428
Fat: 34g
Protein: 21g
Sodium: 625mg
Fiber: 1g
Carbohydrates: 5g
Net Carbohydrates: 4g
Sugar: 2g

1 Preheat oven to 350°F.

2 In a medium bowl, whisk eggs and heavy cream together and set aside.

3 In a medium skillet over medium-high heat, heat olive oil and add vegetables. Sauté vegetables until soft and spinach is wilted, 3–4 minutes.

4 Add vegetables, pepper, salt, and garlic powder to egg mixture and whisk together.

5 Butter the bottom of two 8-ounce custard dishes and sprinkle ⅛ cup of each cheese evenly along bottom of both dishes. Pour equal parts of egg mixture over cheese and sprinkle remaining cheeses on top.

6 Bake 15 minutes or until egg is set.

MAKE IT "MUFFINS"

If you prefer to take this quiche on the go for the busy weekday mornings, you can make it more travel friendly by pouring an equal amount of the egg mixture into four wells of a regular-sized muffin tin. Bake for the same amount of time, allow to cool slightly, and then just grab and go. You can even make them the night before and store them in the refrigerator for the next morning.

BACON HASH (*pictured*)

SERVES 2

This Bacon Hash can be a fat-rich complement to any main dish or you can turn it into a complete meal itself by adding a couple of poached or over-easy eggs on top. You can also mix this Bacon Hash into some scrambled eggs and add some avocado slices.

3 slices no-sugar-added bacon

1 cup chopped cauliflower

½ medium onion, peeled and diced

1 clove garlic, minced

¼ teaspoon salt

¼ teaspoon black pepper

¼ teaspoon garlic powder

1 In a medium skillet over medium heat, cook bacon until crispy, about 10 minutes. Remove from pan and let cool, then dice.

2 Add cauliflower, onion, and garlic to the skillet. Cook 5 minutes over medium heat or until cauliflower starts to brown. Add salt, pepper, garlic powder, and diced bacon. Stir until combined.

3 Remove from heat and serve.

PER SERVING

Calories: 92
Fat: 5g
Protein: 7g
Sodium: 550mg

Fiber: 2g
Carbohydrates: 6g
Net Carbohydrates: 4g
Sugar: 2g

EGG AND MASCARPONE PROSCIUTTO CUPS

SERVES 2

If you want to start your macronutrient ratios off on the right foot, these Egg and Mascarpone Prosciutto Cups are the perfect way to do it. They require only three simple ingredients, and you can sit down together and eat them or take them with you on the go.

4 (0.5-ounce) slices prosciutto

4 large eggs

2 tablespoons mascarpone cheese

1 Preheat oven to 350°F. Use a muffin tin with cups about 2½" wide and 1½" deep.

2 Fold prosciutto slices in half so they become almost square. Place each folded slice in a muffin tin cup to line it completely.

3 Break eggs into prosciutto cups.

4 Gently place mascarpone on top of eggs.

5 Bake about 12 minutes until egg whites are cooked and yolks are still runny but warm.

6 Let cool 10 minutes before removing from muffin tin.

PER SERVING

Calories: 268
Fat: 19g
Protein: 20g
Sodium: 262mg

Fiber: 0g
Carbohydrates: 3g
Net Carbohydrates: 1g
Sugar: 1g

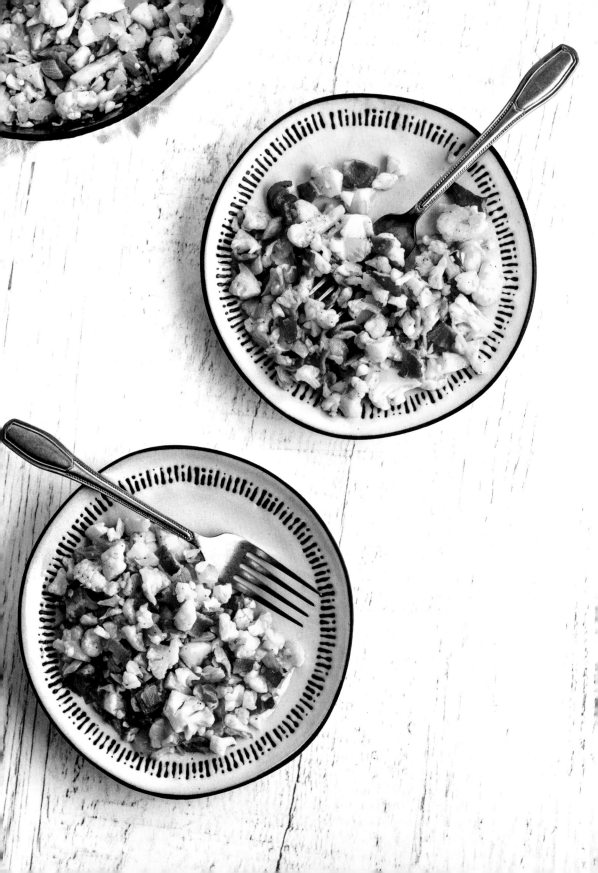

EGG, SOUR CREAM, AND CHIVE BACON CUPS

SERVES 2

Sour cream is an excellent way to add extra fat to your meals and it makes your scrambled eggs taste even creamier. If you'd rather serve this as a sit-down meal for two, you can bake it in 6-ounce quiche cups instead of a muffin tin.

4 slices no-sugar-added bacon, 2 cut in half

4 large eggs

¼ teaspoon salt

¼ teaspoon black pepper

1 tablespoon diced chives

1 tablespoon sour cream

PER SERVING

Calories: 170
Fat: 11g
Protein: 14g
Sodium: 688mg
Fiber: 0g
Carbohydrates: 1g
Net Carbohydrates: 1g
Sugar: 0g

1 Preheat oven to 400°F.

2 In a standard-sized muffin tin, place half strips of bacon in an X shape in the bottom of two cups. Line those same cups with one full slice bacon along the inside of the cup vertically.

3 Place a baking sheet underneath muffin tin and bake cups 8–10 minutes until they're a little pliable.

4 While cups are precooking, in a medium bowl, whisk eggs with remaining ingredients. Set aside.

5 Take muffin tin out of oven and divide egg mixture equally between cups.

6 Bake cups 8–10 minutes more until eggs set. Serve warm.

WESTERN SCRAMBLED EGGS

SERVES 2

If you have some room for some extra fat in your macros and you want to turn up the heat on this scramble, add some chopped avocado and a drizzle of Tessemae's Habanero Ranch on top of the eggs after you put them on a plate.

4 large eggs

2 tablespoons heavy cream

½ teaspoon salt

¼ teaspoon black pepper

½ tablespoon grass-fed butter

¼ cup diced no-sugar-added ham

¼ cup chopped yellow onion

¼ cup chopped red and green bell peppers

½ cup shredded Cheddar cheese

1 tablespoon chopped green onion

1 In a large mixing bowl, whisk eggs, heavy cream, salt, and black pepper together.

2 In a medium skillet over medium heat, melt butter. Add egg mixture and stir. When eggs start to scramble, add ham, onion, and bell peppers. Continue to stir until eggs are almost cooked. Add cheese and stir until eggs are finished cooking, about 30 more seconds.

3 Garnish with green onions and serve.

PER SERVING
Calories: 377
Fat: 27g
Protein: 24g
Sodium: 1,161mg
Fiber: 1g
Carbohydrates: 5g
Net Carbohydrates: 4g
Sugar: 2g

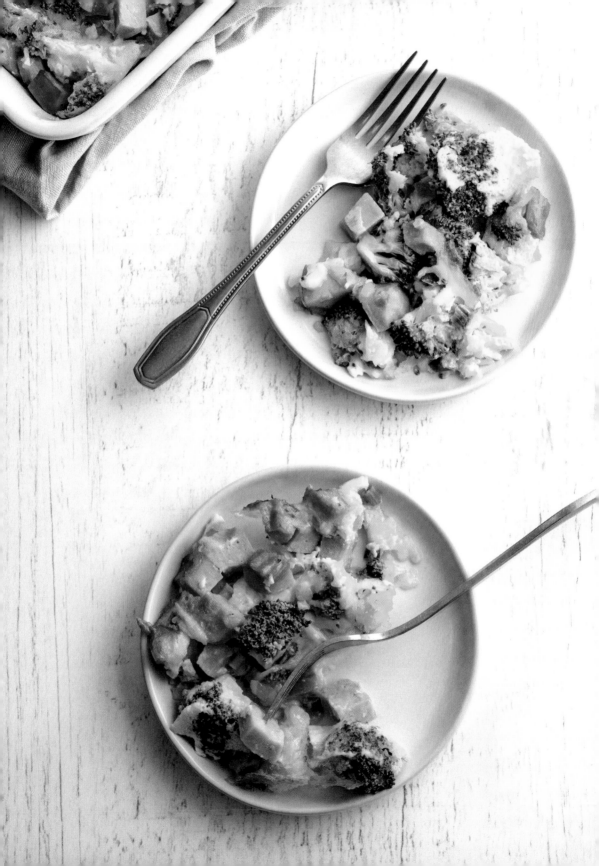

HAM, CHEESE, AND EGG CASSEROLE

SERVES 2

Mozzarella and Cheddar cheeses give this dish a mild cheesy flavor, but you can use any type of shredded cheese you want. If you're choosing prepackaged cheese, check the ingredient list to make sure it falls within your carbohydrate allotment. Some added ingredients can up the carb count.

⅔ cup broccoli florets

2 large eggs

⅔ cup cooked diced sugar-free ham

3 tablespoons shredded mozzarella cheese

3 tablespoons shredded Cheddar cheese

2 teaspoons chopped green onion

1 Preheat oven to 375°F.

2 Fill a large pot with water and bring to a boil. Blanch broccoli by putting in boiling water, 2–3 minutes.

3 In a large bowl, add eggs, ham, mozzarella, Cheddar, and green onions and whisk until combined. Add broccoli.

4 Pour into a 5" × 5" baking pan and cook 20 minutes or until eggs are cooked through.

PER SERVING

Calories: 232
Fat: 13g
Protein: 23g
Sodium: 851mg
Fiber: 1g
Carbohydrates: 3g
Net Carbohydrates: 2g
Sugar: 1g

BUNCHES OF BROCCOLI

One cup of chopped broccoli contains only 6 grams of carbohydrates, half of which come from fiber. At 3 grams of net carbohydrates per cup, it's the perfect green vegetable addition to breakfast, lunch, or dinner. But it's not just the fact that it's low in carbohydrates that makes it impressive; broccoli is also high in vitamin C, a nutrient that you need more of when following a ketogenic diet.

CHAPTER 3

SOUPS AND SALADS

Who doesn't love a hearty soup and a satisfying, healthy fat-filled salad? The recipes in this chapter are simple enough to prepare for a quick lunch, but filling enough to enjoy during a sit-down dinner for two. You'll find everything from Bacon and Broccoli Salad and Avocado and Egg Salad to Pumpkin Cream Soup and a basic Chicken Soup that you can play around with to make your own.

Soups and salads are an excellent way to use up any leftover low-carb veggies so you can reduce the amount of food you waste and stretch your food budget a little further. If you want to take your salads on the go or prepare them in advance, you can make them in glass Mason jars and store them in the refrigerator until you're ready to eat.

BACON CHEDDAR SOUP

SERVES 2

If you don't have an immersion blender, you can pour the soup into the pitcher of a regular blender instead and blend until smooth. Just make sure to let it cool down a little bit. If you put it in the blender when it's too hot, you may have an explosive mess on your hands.

2 slices thick-cut no-sugar-added bacon

½ small yellow onion, peeled and chopped

1 clove garlic, minced

1½ cups cauliflower florets

¼ teaspoon dry mustard

¼ teaspoon black pepper

1½ cups no-sugar-added chicken broth

1 cup heavy cream

1 cup shredded Cheddar cheese

2 teaspoons grated Parmesan cheese

PER SERVING

Calories: 806
Fat: 69g
Protein: 23g
Sodium: 1,348mg
Fiber: 2g
Carbohydrates: 12g
Net Carbohydrates: 10g
Sugar: 7g

1 In a medium skillet over medium-high heat, cook bacon until crisp, about 10 minutes. Remove bacon from pan, reserving bacon grease. Return pan to heat.

2 Place onions and garlic in bacon grease and sauté until translucent, 3–4 minutes. Chop cauliflower florets into small pieces and add to onions and garlic. Sauté until tender, 7–10 minutes. Add dry mustard and pepper and stir.

3 Transfer onions, garlic, cauliflower, and bacon grease to a large stockpot. Add chicken broth and heavy cream.

4 Stir stockpot contents together and bring to a boil over medium heat. Once mixture begins to boil, reduce heat to a simmer.

5 Insert an immersion blender into the soup and blend until creamy. Add Cheddar cheese and Parmesan cheese and stir until melted.

6 Dice bacon and stir into soup. Serve hot.

HOMEMADE CHICKEN BROTH

Many commercial chicken broths contain unhealthy ingredients and preservatives, and while homemade chicken broth doesn't last as long, it's better for you. If you can't find a store-bought chicken broth without added sugar, you can easily make your own by covering about 3 pounds of chicken bones with water in a slow cooker and letting it simmer on low for at least 12 hours.

CREAMY BROCCOLI SOUP

SERVES 2

The coconut milk in this recipe adds a nutty and slightly sweet undertone to the soup that complements the bitterness of the broccoli nicely. However, if you prefer your savory dishes without that hint of coconut, you can use heavy cream in its place.

1 tablespoon grass-fed butter

1 medium stalk celery, diced

¼ cup diced yellow onion

2 cups broccoli florets

¼ teaspoon salt

¼ teaspoon black pepper

1½ cups no-sugar-added chicken broth

½ cup full-fat canned coconut milk

PER SERVING
Calories: 219
Fat: 17g
Protein: 5g
Sodium: 1,054mg
Fiber: 3g
Carbohydrates: 11g
Net Carbohydrates: 8g
Sugar: 3g

1 In a large stockpot over medium-high heat, heat butter. Add celery and onion and sauté until translucent, 3–4 minutes.

2 Add broccoli florets, salt, pepper, and chicken broth and bring to a simmer. Allow to simmer until broccoli is fork tender, about 10 minutes.

3 Add coconut milk and blend with an immersion blender until soup is smooth and creamy. Serve hot.

BE CHOOSY WITH DAIRY

Certain dairy products, including cheeses and heavy cream, can help you meet your macronutrient needs when following a keto diet, but it's best to choose grass-fed versions whenever possible. Grass-fed products not only have higher amounts of CLA and omega fatty acids, they also tend to have a richer, creamier taste and are less inflammatory than dairy products that come from conventional cows who eat mostly grains.

PUMPKIN CREAM SOUP

SERVES 2

You don't have to wait for fall to enjoy this hearty meal for two. Grab a can of pumpkin purée (but not pumpkin pie filling!) and make it any time of the year. To save a little time, instead of using cinnamon, nutmeg, and ginger in this recipe, you can add a couple dashes of pumpkin pie spice instead.

1 tablespoon coconut oil

1 tablespoon grass-fed butter

2 tablespoons minced yellow onion

1 clove garlic, minced

1 cup no-sugar-added chicken broth

½ cup pumpkin purée

¼ teaspoon ground cinnamon

¹⁄₁₆ teaspoon ground nutmeg

¹⁄₁₆ teaspoon ground ginger

⅛ teaspoon salt

⅛ teaspoon black pepper

1 cup full-fat canned coconut milk

1 In a large stockpot over medium-high heat, heat coconut oil and butter. When oil and butter are hot, add onions and garlic and sauté until translucent, 3–4 minutes.

2 Add chicken broth, pumpkin purée, cinnamon, nutmeg, ginger, salt, and pepper and stir until combined.

3 Submerge an immersion blender into soup and blend until smooth and creamy. Allow to simmer for 20 minutes.

4 Stir in coconut milk. Serve hot.

PER SERVING
Calories: 374
Fat: 35g
Protein: 4g
Sodium: 641mg
Fiber: 2g
Carbohydrates: 11g
Net Carbohydrates: 9g
Sugar: 3g

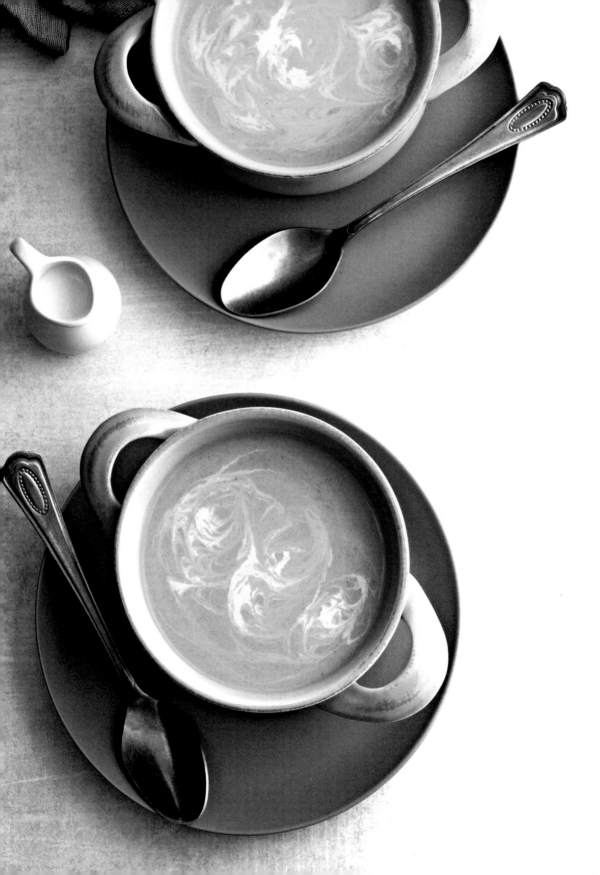

CHICKEN SOUP

SERVES 2

Canned chicken makes this soup easy to whip up in under half an hour. If you don't want to use canned chicken, you can still keep it simple by using the meat from a precooked rotisserie chicken or you can poach a couple of chicken breasts and then shred them.

1 tablespoon olive oil

1 clove garlic, minced

¼ cup diced yellow onion

1 medium stalk celery, diced

2 ounces cream cheese

¼ cup heavy cream

1 (5-ounce) can shredded chicken breast

2 cups no-sugar-added chicken broth

¼ teaspoon dried oregano

¾ teaspoon Italian seasoning

1 bay leaf

1 tablespoon fresh chopped parsley

1 In a large stockpot over medium-high heat, heat olive oil. When oil is hot, add garlic and onions and sauté until translucent, 3–4 minutes. Add celery and sauté until soft, about 4 minutes.

2 Add cream cheese and heavy cream and stir until cream cheese is melted.

3 Add remaining ingredients and bring to a boil. Once the soup starts boiling, reduce heat and allow to simmer for 20 minutes. Remove bay leaf and serve hot.

PER SERVING

Calories: 402
Fat: 30g
Protein: 20g
Sodium: 1,356mg
Fiber: 1g
Carbohydrates: 7g
Net Carbohydrates: 6g
Sugar: 4g

TOMATO CREAM SOUP

SERVES 2

You can finish this Tomato Cream Soup off with a dollop of sour cream, which, in addition to adding a nice creamy texture to each spoonful, also ups the fat content a little bit.

¼ cup grass-fed butter

½ medium yellow onion, peeled and diced

1 clove garlic, minced

1 (14.5-ounce) can whole peeled tomatoes

1½ cups no-sugar-added vegetable broth

½ cup full-fat coconut milk

2 tablespoons chopped fresh basil

2 tablespoons chopped fresh parsley

¼ teaspoon salt

⅛ teaspoon black pepper

1 In a medium stockpot over medium-high heat, heat butter. Add onion and garlic and sauté until translucent, 3–4 minutes.

2 Add remaining ingredients and stir until combined.

3 Insert an immersion blender and blend all ingredients together until smooth.

4 Turn heat to high and bring to a boil. Once soup starts boiling, reduce heat and allow to simmer for 30 minutes. Serve hot.

PER SERVING

Calories: 404
Fat: 35g
Protein: 2g
Sodium: 1,618mg
Fiber: 2g
Carbohydrates: 19g
Net Carbohydrates: 17g
Sugar: 13g

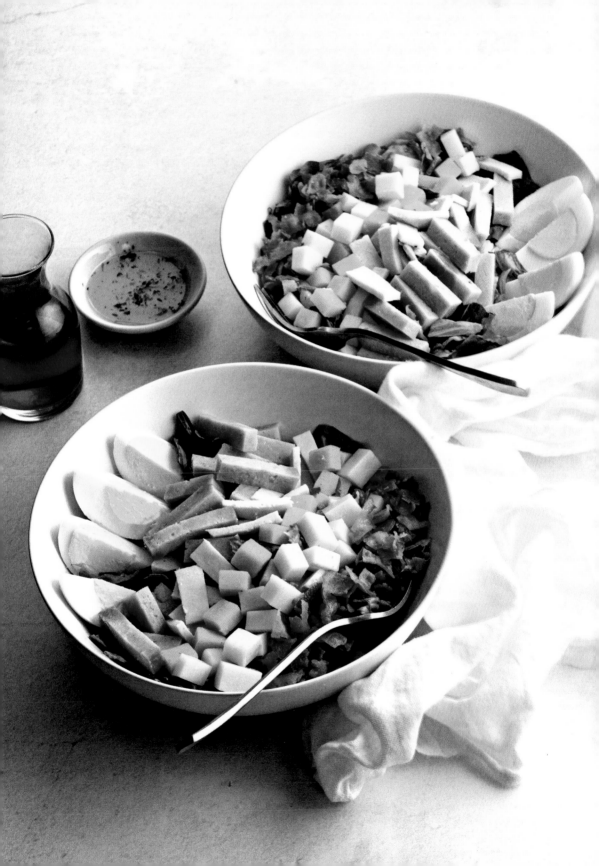

CHEF SALAD (pictured)

SERVES 2

Meat and cheese are the basis of a chef salad. Although this recipe calls for ham and turkey and Swiss and Cheddar, you can use any combination you'd like. Try adding roast beef and some pepper jack for a little kick. Drizzle some keto-friendly Avocado Ranch dressing from Tessemae's on top to complete the meal.

4 cups chopped romaine lettuce

½ cup diced no-sugar-added ham

½ cup diced turkey

½ cup cubed Swiss cheese

½ cup cubed Cheddar cheese

2 large hard-boiled eggs, sliced

¼ cup crumbled no-sugar-added bacon

Combine all ingredients in a large bowl and toss to combine. Serve immediately.

PER SERVING

Calories: 581	Fiber: 2g
Fat: 35g	Carbohydrates: 7g
Protein: 50g	Net Carbohydrates: 5g
Sodium: 1,340mg	Sugar: 2g

COLESLAW

SERVES 2

This Coleslaw is a quick and easy fat addition to your bunless burgers or any main protein source. If you want to switch it up, you can use shredded broccoli slaw, which only contains 3 grams of net carbohydrates per serving, in place of the cabbage.

3 tablespoons keto-friendly mayonnaise

1 tablespoon sour cream

½ tablespoon white vinegar

¼ teaspoon celery salt

⅛ teaspoon black pepper

2 teaspoons granulated erythritol

2 cups shredded green cabbage

2 teaspoons chopped yellow onion

1 In a large bowl, combine mayonnaise, sour cream, vinegar, celery salt, pepper, and granulated erythritol and whisk until combined and the granulated erythritol is dissolved.

2 Add cabbage and onion to bowl and toss until coated.

3 Refrigerate 30 minutes. Serve chilled.

PER SERVING

Calories: 179	Fiber: 2g
Fat: 19g	Carbohydrates: 8g
Protein: 1g	Net Carbohydrates: 4g
Sodium: 272mg	Sugar: 0g

SPINACH AND TUNA SALAD

SERVES 2

You can swap out the tuna for chicken in this salad or add hard-boiled eggs for some variations in taste. Make it spicy by adding a pinch of cayenne pepper or a dash of keto-friendly hot sauce, like Tessemae's or The New Primal.

1 (5-ounce) can tuna, packed in water

2 medium stalks celery, diced

3 tablespoons keto-friendly mayonnaise

4 cups spinach

4 slices sugar-free bacon, cooked and crumbled

1 large avocado, peeled, pitted, and diced

2 tablespoons extra-virgin olive oil

¼ teaspoon freshly ground black pepper

1 In a small bowl, combine tuna, celery, and mayonnaise and mix until combined.

2 In a large bowl, mix spinach, bacon crumbles, and avocado. Top with tuna mixture, drizzle with olive oil, and add pepper. Serve immediately.

MERCURY CONCERNS

If you're concerned about the mercury in tuna, keep in mind that adults can safely eat 18–24 ounces of tuna per month without a significant amount of mercury getting into their systems. If you'd like, swap out the tuna for canned salmon. Canned salmon is higher in omega-3 fatty acids and contains no mercury.

PER SERVING
Calories: 582
Fat: 50g
Protein: 25g
Sodium: 611mg
Fiber: 7g
Carbohydrates: 10g
Net Carbohydrates: 3g
Sugar: 1g

AVOCADO AND EGG SALAD

SERVES 2

Instead of mashing the avocado into the salad along with the mayonnaise, you can cut it up into big chunks and toss it to cover with mayonnaise.

3 large hard-boiled eggs

2 tablespoons keto-friendly mayonnaise

½ medium avocado, peeled, pitted, and chopped

¼ teaspoon dried minced onion

¼ teaspoon salt

⅛ teaspoon black pepper

⅛ teaspoon dry mustard powder

PER SERVING

Calories: 264
Fat: 23g
Protein: 10g
Sodium: 474mg
Fiber: 2g
Carbohydrates: 4g
Net Carbohydrates: 2g
Sugar: 0g

1 Peel eggs and put into a medium mixing bowl. Mash eggs with a fork.

2 Add mayonnaise and avocado and continue to mash with a fork until combined. Stir in minced onion, salt, pepper, and dry mustard powder.

A HEALTHY DOSE OF FAT

A single avocado contains 29 grams of fat, 75 percent of which are in the form of unsaturated fats. The monounsaturated fats in avocados have been shown to help promote weight loss, decrease inflammation, and reduce the risk of heart disease. With a creamy, neutral taste and only 4 grams of net carbohydrates for a whole avocado, they make an excellent fat addition to almost any meal.

BACON AND BROCCOLI SALAD

SERVES 2

With a low carb count, green vegetable, and four different fat sources, this Bacon and Broccoli Salad is the perfect keto side dish for two. As this recipe chills in the refrigerator, the flavors meld together, so the longer it sits, the better it gets. If you remember, make it the night before you plan to eat it for maximum flavor.

3 cups broccoli florets

4 slices no-sugar-added bacon, cooked and crumbled

4 ounces sharp Cheddar cheese, cubed

½ large avocado, peeled, pitted, and diced

½ cup keto-friendly mayonnaise

1 tablespoon white vinegar

¼ teaspoon salt

¼ teaspoon black pepper

2 teaspoons powdered erythritol

PER SERVING
Calories: 881
Fat: 80g
Protein: 26g
Sodium: 1,392mg
Fiber: 8g
Carbohydrates: 18g
Net Carbohydrates: 8g
Sugar: 3g

1 In a large bowl, combine broccoli, bacon, Cheddar cheese, and avocado.

2 In a separate small bowl, combine mayonnaise, vinegar, salt, pepper, and erythritol and stir until combined. Pour dressing over broccoli mixture and toss to coat. Refrigerate until chilled, about 30 minutes. Serve chilled.

GO RAW

Broccoli contains a high amount of sulforaphane, a compound that helps stimulate detoxification and may help reduce the risk for certain types of cancers. According to a report in the *Journal of Agricultural and Food Chemistry*, raw broccoli provides more sulforaphane than cooked broccoli, because the cooking process binds the compounds, making it less accessible.

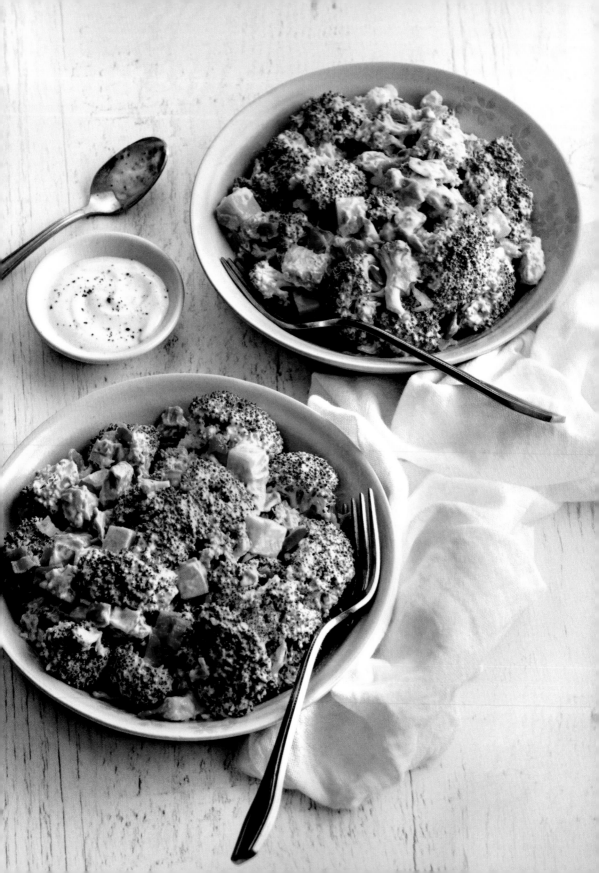

CHAPTER 4

APPETIZERS AND SNACKS

Although people generally view appetizers and snacks in a negative light, they can be vital to helping you stay on track with your keto plan. Most commercial snack foods are high in sugar, salt, and artificial ingredients. While you want to stay away from those, these keto-approved appetizers and snacks not only help you curb your hunger and cravings in between meals; they also offer balanced macronutrients and vitamins and minerals that contribute to your health, instead of detracting from it.

Of course, when snacking, you have to watch your portions, but since these recipes are all perfectly designed for two, overeating and overindulging isn't really an issue. With everything from Crab Rangoon Dip and Pizza Bites to Meaty Zucchini Balls with Yogurt Sauce, this chapter has your back.

BACON OLIVE SPREAD

SERVES 2

This Bacon Olive Spread is great served on celery sticks or cucumber slices—two vegetables that add maximum crunch but only a minimal amount of carbs. If you don't have Spanish olives, you can use black ones in their place for a milder flavor. Serve it immediately or make it the night before and let it chill in the refrigerator before serving.

2 slices no-sugar-added bacon

4 ounces cream cheese, softened

1 tablespoon keto-friendly mayonnaise

1½ teaspoons freshly squeezed lemon juice

12 Spanish olives, sliced

PER SERVING
Calories: 320
Fat: 29g
Protein: 7g
Sodium: 689mg
Fiber: 1g
Carbohydrates: 3g
Net Carbohydrates: 2g
Sugar: 2g

1 In a large skillet over medium heat, cook bacon until crisp, 5 minutes per side. Drain on a paper towel.

2 In a medium mixing bowl, beat cream cheese with a hand mixer until smooth.

3 Add mayonnaise and lemon juice and mix on medium speed until combined.

4 Crumble bacon into bowl followed by sliced olives. Fold bacon and olives into cream cheese mixture by hand with rubber spatula. Serve.

CRAB RANGOON DIP

SERVES 2

Following a keto diet doesn't mean you can't enjoy the same flavors of your favorite Chinese takeout. This Crab Rangoon Dip offers all the creamy goodness of the real thing, but without the added carbohydrates. Enjoy it on celery sticks or Parmesan crisps on your next date night.

4 ounces cream cheese, softened

1 tablespoon keto-friendly mayonnaise

1½ teaspoons freshly squeezed lemon juice

⅛ teaspoon sea salt

⅛ teaspoon black pepper

1 clove garlic, minced

1 green onion, diced

¼ cup shredded Parmesan cheese

2 ounces canned white crabmeat

PER SERVING
Calories: 324
Fat: 26g
Protein: 12g
Sodium: 717mg
Fiber: 0g
Carbohydrates: 5g
Net Carbohydrates: 5g
Sugar: 2g

1 Preheat oven to 350°F.

2 In a medium bowl, mix cream cheese, mayonnaise, lemon juice, salt, and pepper with a hand blender until well incorporated.

3 Add garlic, onions, Parmesan, and crabmeat and fold into mixture with a spatula.

4 Transfer mixture to an oven-safe crock and spread out evenly.

5 Bake 25–30 minutes or until top of dip is slightly browned. Serve warm.

ALLICIN AND ALLIUM

Like shallots, garlic belongs to the genus *Allium*, which also includes onions and leeks. The major compound in garlic, which is called allicin, is responsible for its smell as well as its health benefits, which include boosting the immune system, lowering blood pressure, and reducing the risk of Alzheimer's disease and dementia.

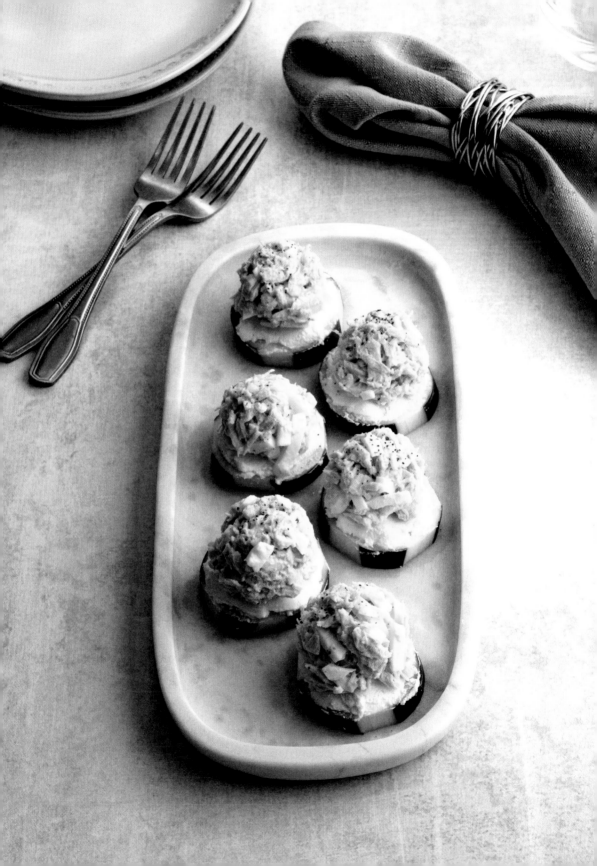

TUNA SALAD AND CUCUMBER BITES

(pictured)

SERVES 2

These Tuna Salad and Cucumber Bites are an easy snack that's good on the go or for a quick picnic for two. Give yourself a little variety by using canned chicken or canned salmon in place of tuna or using raw zucchini slices in place of the cucumber.

1 (5-ounce) can tuna packed in water

1 large hard-boiled egg, chopped

¼ cup keto-friendly mayonnaise

¼ teaspoon salt

¼ teaspoon black pepper

1 tablespoon goat cheese

½ medium cucumber, cut into rounds

1 Drain tuna and put in a medium bowl with chopped eggs, mayonnaise, salt, and pepper. Mash with a fork until combined.

2 Spread an equal amount of goat cheese on each cucumber slice and top with tuna salad mixture. Serve.

PER SERVING

Calories: 349
Fat: 30g
Protein: 19g
Sodium: 324mg

Fiber: 0g
Carbohydrates: 3g
Net Carbohydrates: 3g
Sugar: 2g

PEPPERONI CHEESE BITES

SERVES 2

String cheese isn't just a childhood favorite. It's also a keto diet snack staple. When you're feeling hungry between meals, you can easily enjoy this quick treat right from the refrigerator. If you have a little extra time, put each Pepperoni Cheese Bite in the oven just until the cheese melts for a warm, tasty treat.

2 sticks mozzarella string cheese

8 slices sugar-free pepperoni

1 Cut each string cheese into four equal pieces.

2 Wrap each piece in one slice pepperoni and secure with a toothpick.

PER SERVING

Calories: 109
Fat: 8g
Protein: 8g
Sodium: 315mg

Fiber: 0g
Carbohydrates: 0g
Net Carbohydrates: 0g
Sugar: 0g

PIZZA BITES

SERVES 2

Pizza is a diet staple, so don't let keto stop you from enjoying a pizza night together. When you try these Pizza Bites, you won't even miss the crust. And the best part? They're ready to go in under 5 minutes, so you can spend less time in the kitchen and more time eating together.

8 slices sugar-free pepperoni

3 tablespoons no-sugar-added marinara sauce

3 tablespoons shredded mozzarella cheese

PER SERVING
Calories: 78
Fat: 5g
Protein: 5g
Sodium: 256mg
Fiber: 0g
Carbohydrates: 2g
Net Carbohydrates: 2g
Sugar: 1g

1 Turn on oven broiler.

2 Line a baking sheet with parchment paper and put pepperoni slices in a single layer on baking sheet.

3 Put equal amounts of marinara sauce on each pepperoni slice and spread out with a spoon. Add equal amounts of cheese on top of marinara.

4 Put baking sheet in the oven and broil 3 minutes or until cheese is melted and slightly brown.

5 Remove from baking sheet and transfer to a paper towel–lined baking sheet to absorb excess grease. Serve warm.

THE PERFECT KETO PIZZA DOUGH

If you want to take these Pizza Bites from an appetizer or snack to a meal, turn them into a keto-approved pie instead. Melt 1 cup shredded mozzarella cheese, ½ cup shredded Cheddar cheese, and 2 ounces cream cheese together in a bowl. Transfer to a food processor and add 1½ cups fine almond flour, 1 large egg, and ¼ teaspoon garlic powder and pulse until a dough forms. Roll out on a parchment paper–lined baking sheet, poke holes in the dough with a fork, bake at 425°F for 8 minutes, and then finish off with no-sugar-added pizza sauce and your favorite toppings and bake again until cheese is melted.

JALAPEÑO POPPERS

SERVES 2

If you want to spice up your date night, whip up a couple of these Jalapeño Poppers for a perfectly balanced keto appetizer. If you prefer to keep things mild, you can use a green bell pepper, which only has 4 net carbohydrates, in place of the jalapeños.

4 medium jalapeño peppers

2 ounces cream cheese, softened

¼ cup shredded pepper jack cheese

4 slices no-sugar-added bacon

PER SERVING

Calories: 267
Fat: 20g
Protein: 13g
Sodium: 577mg
Fiber: 1g
Carbohydrates: 3g
Net Carbohydrates: 2g
Sugar: 2g

1 Preheat oven to 425°F. Line a baking sheet with aluminum foil.

2 Cut each pepper in half lengthwise. Scoop out seeds.

3 In a small bowl, mix together cream cheese and pepper jack cheese. Divide filling into four equal portions and stuff each pepper with cheese filling.

4 Wrap each pepper in bacon. Lay flat on baking sheet and bake 15–20 minutes, or until bacon is crispy.

TURN UP THE HEAT

The capsaicin in chili peppers is thermogenic, which means it generates heat by increasing the metabolism of your adipose, or fat, tissue. Eating capsaicin-rich foods, like jalapeños, may help stimulate the body's ability to burn fat. If you're not a fan of jalapeños, you can boost your capsaicin intake by adding cayenne pepper or red pepper flakes to your favorite dishes for some extra heat and fat-burning potential.

STUFFED BABY BELLA MUSHROOM CAPS

SERVES 2

Sometimes it's difficult to find breakfast sausage without any added sugar at big box grocery stores. Try going to a local farm or butcher and asking them to whip up a batch of keto-friendly pork sausage for you instead. If you don't have one near you, you can make your own or just use plain ground pork instead.

½ tablespoon olive oil

4 baby bella mushrooms, cleaned and stems removed

⅛ teaspoon salt

2 ounces no-sugar-added pork breakfast sausage, at room temperature

2 tablespoons chopped fresh parsley

¼ cup shredded Parmesan cheese

1 Preheat oven to 350°F.

2 Rub olive oil on mushroom tops and sprinkle lightly with salt.

3 In a small bowl, mix sausage, parsley, and cheese.

4 Stuff each mushroom cap until mixture forms a nice cap slightly above the mushroom ribbing.

5 Bake on a baking sheet roughly 20 minutes until sausage becomes browned and cheese browns slightly. Serve warm.

PER SERVING
Calories: 178
Fat: 13g
Protein: 10g
Sodium: 660mg
Fiber: 0g
Carbohydrates: 4g
Net Carbohydrates: 4g
Sugar: 1g

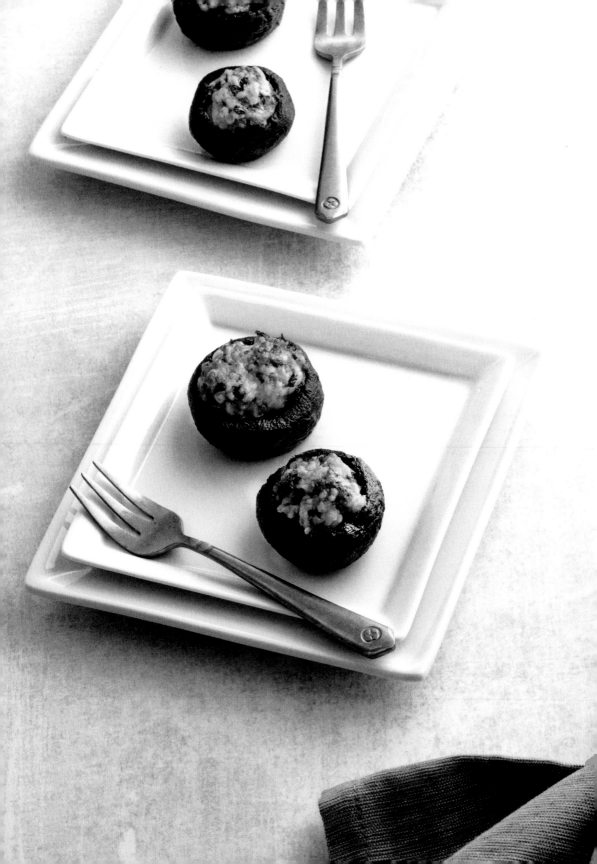

MONKEY SALAD

SERVES 2

Traditional monkey salad uses sliced bananas as a base, and that's where the "monkey" name comes from. Because bananas are high in carbohydrates, this version leaves them out, but the flavor is so good, you won't even miss them.

1 tablespoon grass-fed butter

¼ cup unsweetened coconut flakes

¼ cup raw unsalted cashews

¼ cup raw unsalted almonds

⅛ cup 90% dark chocolate shavings

PER SERVING
Calories: 366
Fat: 32g
Protein: 8g
Sodium: 5mg
Fiber: 5g
Carbohydrates: 15g
Net Carbohydrates: 10g
Sugar: 3g

1 In a medium skillet over medium heat, melt butter. Add coconut flakes and sauté until lightly browned, 3–4 minutes.

2 Add cashews and almonds and sauté for 2 minutes. Remove from heat and sprinkle with dark chocolate shavings. Serve immediately.

A SWEET TREAT

Monkey Salad is the perfect sweet and satisfying treat. It's loaded with healthy fats that help keep you full between meals, but the dark chocolate gives it just the right amount of sweetness to curb any sugar cravings. It's also easy to take on the go, so you can make it in the morning or the night before you need a portable snack for the two of you.

PARMESAN VEGETABLE CRISPS

SERVES 2

This simple twist on the Parmesan crisp introduces added texture and a mild sweetness while offering additional fiber too. If neither of you eat carrots on your keto plan, you can replace the carrots with more zucchini instead to lower the carb count slightly. Enjoy these crisps as is or with other fat-bomb dips and spreads.

¾ cup shredded zucchini

¼ cup shredded carrots

1 cup freshly shredded Parmesan cheese

1 tablespoon olive oil

¼ teaspoon black pepper

PER SERVING

Calories: 238
Fat: 17g
Protein: 16g
Sodium: 690mg
Fiber: 1g
Carbohydrates: 4g
Net Carbohydrates: 3g
Sugar: 2g

1 Preheat oven to 375°F. Prepare a baking sheet with parchment paper or a Silpat mat.

2 Wrap shredded vegetables in a paper towel and wring out excess moisture.

3 In a medium bowl, mix all ingredients together until thoroughly combined.

4 Place tablespoon-sized mounds onto prepared baking sheet.

5 Bake 7–10 minutes until lightly browned.

6 Let cool 2–3 minutes and remove from mat. Serve.

ZUCCHINI: A KITCHEN STAPLE

It's no secret that the right vegetables are an important part of any healthy diet. Zucchini is a fantastic choice for a keto diet because it has a low carbohydrate content (low glycemic index) and it's full of potassium, a crucial mineral for heart health. Besides that, it also makes a fantastic substitute for pasta lovers looking for low-carbohydrate alternatives.

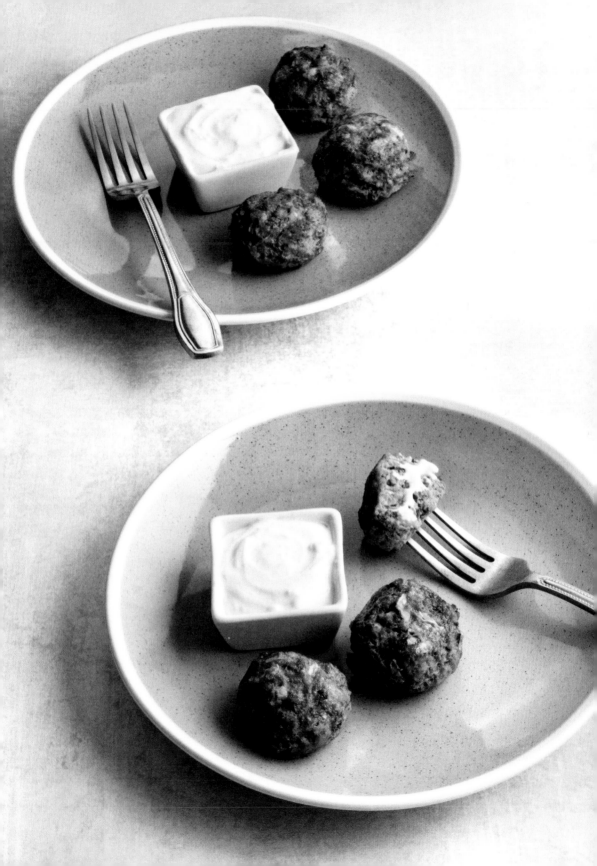

MEATY ZUCCHINI BALLS WITH YOGURT SAUCE

SERVES 2

These meatballs take on a refreshing flavor with the omission of bread crumbs and the use of bright and flavorful zucchini and mint. Adding a yogurt sauce gives them an added Mediterranean flair and a little more fat. If regular yogurt has too many carbs for you, you can replace it with more sour cream instead.

FOR YOGURT SAUCE

2 tablespoons sour cream

2½ tablespoons plain full-fat Greek yogurt

¼ tablespoon lemon juice

½ clove garlic, minced

½ tablespoon olive oil

⅛ teaspoon salt

FOR MEATBALLS

1 large egg

¼ pound 80/20 ground chuck

½ medium zucchini, grated

1 green onion, thinly sliced

½ tablespoon chopped fresh mint leaves

½ tablespoon chopped fresh basil

½ clove garlic, minced

¼ teaspoon paprika

¼ teaspoon salt

⅛ teaspoon cayenne pepper

⅛ teaspoon black pepper

½ tablespoon coconut oil

1 Preheat oven to 350°F.

2 In a small bowl, mix all ingredients for yogurt sauce. Chill at least 1 hour.

3 In a separate small bowl, whisk egg for meatballs. In a medium bowl, mix remaining meatball ingredients thoroughly, adding whisked egg last to bind.

4 Form meat mixture into six equal balls and place into a muffin tin. Place tin on top of a baking sheet and put in oven.

5 Bake meatballs 30 minutes or until meat is browned and internal temperature is at least 165°F.

6 Serve warm with yogurt sauce to dip.

PER SERVING

Calories: 231
Fat: 15g
Protein: 16g
Sodium: 522mg
Fiber: 1g
Carbohydrates: 4g
Net Carbohydrates: 3g
Sugar: 3g

CHAPTER 5

SIDE DISHES

When you're in doubt about what to eat for dinner, it's easy to throw some burgers on the grill or bake a couple of chicken thighs in the oven, but it can be difficult to figure out how to make keto-approved side dishes that are more exciting than plain cauliflower rice or steamed broccoli. Luckily, this chapter has you covered.

Need some keto "Mac" 'n' Cheese for two? You'll find it here (and you'll be pleasantly surprised at how simple it is to make). Looking for some Cheesy Bacon Brussels Sprouts instead? You'll find those here too, and they'll change your mind for good about Brussels sprouts.

Side dishes don't have to be complicated to be satisfying. After trying the recipes in this chapter, you'll be surprised at how combining simple ingredients in the right ways can transform ordinary vegetables into something incredible.

"MAC" 'N' CHEESE

SERVES 2

Of course, there's no real "mac" in this "Mac" 'n' Cheese, but low-carbohydrate cauliflower provides a hearty substitute that makes it hard to miss the pasta. You can turn this comfort food favorite into a vegetarian option by simply omitting the crushed pork rinds, which add a nice texture, but aren't totally necessary.

2 cups cauliflower florets

1 ounce cream cheese

⅓ cup heavy cream

½ cup shredded Cheddar cheese, divided

¼ teaspoon black pepper

⅛ teaspoon garlic powder

¼ teaspoon salt

2 tablespoons crushed pork rinds

PER SERVING
Calories: 356
Fat: 28g
Protein: 14g
Sodium: 656mg
Fiber: 2g
Carbohydrates: 8g
Net Carbohydrates: 6g
Sugar: 4g

1 Preheat oven to 375°F.

2 Fill a double boiler with water and bring water to a boil. Cut cauliflower into small pieces and place in the top portion of the double boiler. Steam until tender, about 5 minutes.

3 Remove cauliflower from double boiler and place in a strainer.

4 In a medium saucepan over medium heat, melt cream cheese. Add heavy cream and whisk until combined. Whisk in ¼ cup Cheddar cheese, pepper, garlic powder, and salt. Once cheese has melted, remove from heat.

5 Transfer strained cauliflower to an 8" × 8" baking pan. Pour in cheese mixture and toss to coat cauliflower. Sprinkle remaining ¼ cup cheese and pork rinds on top. Bake until bubbly, about 20 minutes.

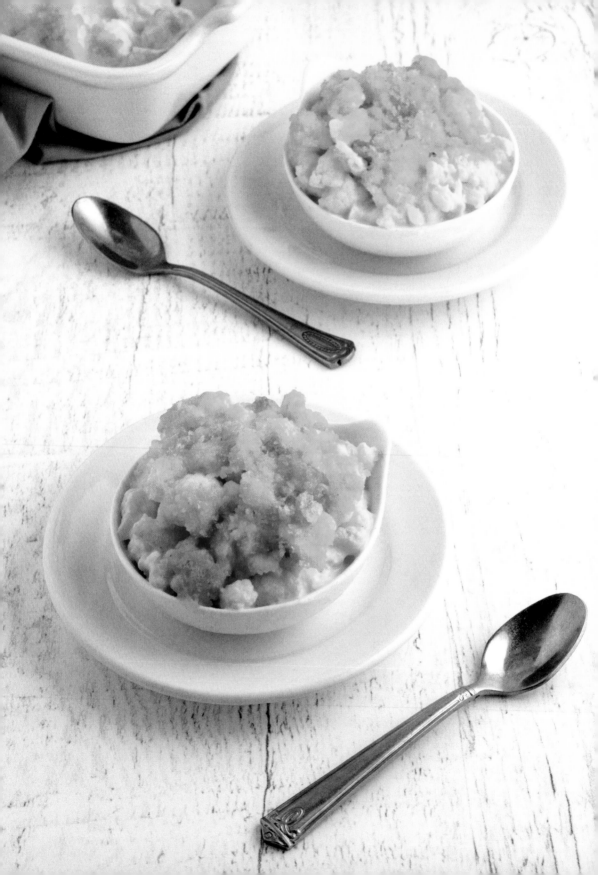

MASHED CAULIFLOWER

SERVES 2

If you need to increase your fat intake for the day, this Mashed Cauliflower is a great way to do it. It hides heavy cream, cream cheese, and grass-fed butter—three keto staples that provide different types of healthy fats. It's also extremely delicious, so fair warning: You're going to have trouble sharing it.

2 cups cauliflower florets

¼ cup heavy cream

2 ounces cream cheese, softened

2 tablespoons grass-fed butter

¼ teaspoon garlic salt

¼ teaspoon salt

¼ teaspoon black pepper

PER SERVING
Calories: 336
Fat: 31g
Protein: 4g
Sodium: 716mg
Fiber: 2g
Carbohydrates: 7g
Net Carbohydrates: 5g
Sugar: 4g

1 Steam cauliflower in a double boiler until fork tender, about 8 minutes.

2 Remove from heat and transfer to a food processor. Add remaining ingredients and process until smooth.

SMOOTH OPERATOR

Using a food processor makes this cauliflower perfectly smooth and creamy and easy to whip together in minutes. If you prefer a chunkier version, use a handheld mixer or an immersion blender instead and stop beating when the cauliflower has reached your desired consistency.

CREAMED BRUSSELS SPROUTS

SERVES 2

For a cheesier, gooier side dish, add ½ cup shredded Cheddar cheese (or any cheese of your choice) to these Creamed Brussels Sprouts before you sprinkle on the pork rinds.

3 tablespoons grass-fed butter, divided

1 clove garlic, minced

1 cup sliced Brussels sprouts

¼ cup heavy cream

1 tablespoon grated Parmesan cheese

⅛ teaspoon salt

⅛ teaspoon black pepper

¼ cup crushed pork rinds

PER SERVING
Calories: 358
Fat: 33g
Protein: 9g
Sodium: 434mg
Fiber: 2g
Carbohydrates: 5g
Net Carbohydrates: 3g
Sugar: 2g

1 Preheat oven to 350°F.

2 In a medium skillet over medium-high heat, heat 2 tablespoons butter. Add garlic and sauté 3 minutes. Add Brussels sprouts and continue to sauté until Brussels sprouts are fork tender, about 5 minutes.

3 Transfer Brussels sprouts, garlic, and melted butter to a 9" × 9" baking pan. Add heavy cream, Parmesan cheese, salt, and pepper. Sprinkle pork rinds evenly over the top of Brussels sprouts and top with remaining 1 tablespoon butter.

4 Cover and bake 30 minutes. Serve hot.

THE BITTERNESS IN BRUSSELS SPROUTS

Brussels sprouts tend to be a vegetable that people either love or hate because of their signature bitter flavor. If you're a Brussels sprouts hater, or cooking for one, you may be able to convert with a few tips. Choose small Brussels sprouts, which tend to be sweeter than larger ones, and ones that are firm and bright green. Once you've got your bunch of Brussels sprouts, cut off the rough stem and outer layers before preparing them for cooking.

FRIED CAULIFLOWER "RICE"

SERVES 2

If you're shredding your own cauliflower, process it just enough to create rice-like pieces, but not so much that it begins to blend together. If you process it too long, it will turn into mashed cauliflower, which is delicious, but not what you want for this recipe.

2 cups cauliflower florets

1 tablespoon grass-fed butter

1 tablespoon sesame oil

2 cloves garlic, minced

1 medium green onion, chopped

2 teaspoons coconut aminos

¼ teaspoon garlic salt

1 large egg, beaten

½ large avocado, peeled, pitted, and sliced

1 Place cauliflower florets into a food processor and process using the grating attachment.

2 In a large wok or skillet, heat butter and sesame oil over medium heat. Add minced garlic and sauté 3 minutes.

3 Add cauliflower and sauté another 5 minutes, stirring frequently, until cauliflower is softened. Add green onion, coconut aminos, garlic salt, and egg and toss until eggs are cooked.

4 Top with sliced avocado and serve.

PER SERVING
Calories: 244
Fat: 20g
Protein: 6g
Sodium: 447mg
Fiber: 5g
Carbohydrates: 11g
Net Carbohydrates: 6g
Sugar: 2g

SKIP THE SOY

Coconut aminos is a soy-free seasoning alternative made from the sap of coconut blossoms that you can use in place of soy sauce in any of your recipes. There is absolutely no coconut flavor—it tastes just like soy sauce, but unlike soy sauce, which is highly processed and most likely contains GMOs, coconut aminos is GMO-free and contains seventeen amino acids, vitamins, and minerals.

BACON-FRIED CABBAGE

SERVES 2

Cabbage comes in several varieties including green, red, and Napa. They're all low in carbohydrates, so for this recipe, you can use any type of cabbage you want. If you're a cabbage newbie, you may want to go for green cabbage, which has a milder flavor than the other varieties.

4 slices no-sugar-added bacon

2 cups chopped green cabbage

2 tablespoons chopped yellow onion

½ teaspoon garlic powder

½ teaspoon black pepper

¼ teaspoon salt

1 In a large skillet over medium-high heat, fry bacon until crispy, about 10 minutes. Remove bacon from heat and set aside. Allow to cool, then roughly chop.

2 Add chopped cabbage and chopped onion to hot bacon fat and sauté until cabbage is tender, about 8 minutes. Add garlic powder, pepper, salt, and chopped bacon to cabbage and toss to combine. Serve.

PER SERVING

Calories: 258
Fat: 21g
Protein: 8g
Sodium: 673mg
Fiber: 2g
Carbohydrates: 7g
Net Carbohydrates: 5g
Sugar: 3g

TURNIP FRIES

SERVES 2

Turnips are often overlooked at the supermarket, but they make a great alternative to carbohydrate-loaded potatoes when making fries. You can also make this recipe with zucchini instead, but the finished product will be less crispy.

2 medium turnips, peeled and cut into 2" sticks

2 tablespoons olive oil

4 tablespoons grated Parmesan cheese

¼ teaspoon salt

¼ teaspoon black pepper

¼ teaspoon chili powder

PER SERVING

Calories: 166
Fat: 12g
Protein: 4g
Sodium: 561mg
Fiber: 2g
Carbohydrates: 10g
Net Carbohydrates: 8g
Sugar: 5g

1 Preheat oven to 425°F.

2 Place turnip sticks on foil-lined baking sheet in a single layer. Sprinkle olive oil, Parmesan cheese, salt, pepper, and chili powder over turnips and toss to coat.

3 Bake 15 minutes, flip fries over, and then bake another 15 minutes. Serve warm.

USING AN AIR FRYER

You can easily convert many recipes that call for oven time into an air fryer recipe. Fries do especially well in the air fryer because the circulating air allows them to crisp up better and faster. If you have an air fryer at home, place your cut turnips in the basket and air-fry at 400°F for 15 minutes or until the fries start to turn slightly golden.

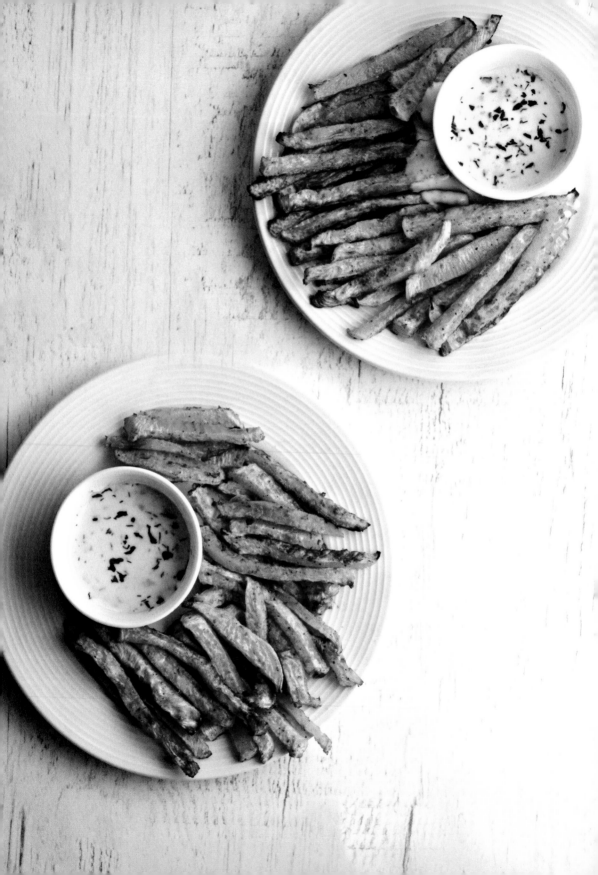

BUTTERY GARLIC SPINACH

SERVES 2

This recipe calls for frozen spinach, but you can use fresh spinach in its place if you prefer. Choose a mature, full-grown spinach instead of baby spinach, which wilts and turns slimy when cooking, and thoroughly clean and chop the leaves before starting the recipe.

2 tablespoons grass-fed butter

1 clove garlic, minced

½ (10-ounce) package frozen spinach, thawed and drained

⅛ teaspoon garlic salt

⅛ teaspoon black pepper

In a medium skillet over medium-high heat, heat butter. Add garlic and sauté 3 minutes. Add spinach and stir until wilted. Toss with garlic salt and pepper. Serve.

PER SERVING

Calories: 132
Fat: 12g
Protein: 3g
Sodium: 209mg
Fiber: 2g
Carbohydrates: 4g
Net Carbohydrates: 2g
Sugar: 0g

CHEESY BROCCOLI

SERVES 2

Instead of using only broccoli, you can make this dish with a combination of broccoli and cauliflower for some variety. If you don't have dry mustard, you can use a teaspoon of regular yellow mustard in its place. Make sure to read the ingredient list to double-check that there isn't any added sugar.

2 cups broccoli florets, fresh or frozen

1 tablespoon extra-virgin olive oil

¼ teaspoon salt

⅛ teaspoon black pepper

1 tablespoon grass-fed butter

½ cup heavy cream

½ cup shredded Cheddar cheese

1 tablespoon grated Asiago cheese

⅛ teaspoon dry mustard

1 Preheat oven to 400°F.

2 Put broccoli florets on a foil-lined baking sheet and toss with olive oil, salt, and pepper. Bake 25 minutes or until broccoli is fork tender.

3 While broccoli is cooking, melt butter in a medium saucepan over medium heat. Add heavy cream and bring to a simmer. Reduce heat to low, add Cheddar cheese and Asiago cheese, and whisk until melted. Stir in dry mustard.

4 Remove from heat and pour over broccoli. Serve.

PER SERVING

Calories: 475
Fat: 43g
Protein: 11g
Sodium: 572mg
Fiber: 2g
Carbohydrates: 8g
Net Carbohydrates: 6g
Sugar: 3g

CREAMED SPINACH

SERVES 2

Creamed Spinach is an easy way to get some low-carb, micronutrient-rich greens in with a healthy dose of fat from butter, cream, and cheese. It goes well with any main protein, so grill up a couple chicken breasts or steaks and serve this on the side.

2 tablespoons grass-fed butter

1 clove garlic, minced

2 tablespoons minced shallots

½ (10-ounce) package frozen spinach, thawed and drained

¼ cup heavy cream

¼ cup grated Parmesan cheese

2 tablespoons grated Asiago cheese

¼ teaspoon salt

⅛ teaspoon black pepper

1 In a medium skillet over medium-high heat, heat butter and add garlic and shallots. Sauté 3 minutes. Add spinach and stir in heavy cream.

2 Stir in Parmesan and Asiago cheeses and continue stirring until melted. Season with salt and pepper. Serve hot.

PER SERVING

Calories: 314
Fat: 27g
Protein: 8g
Sodium: 675mg
Fiber: 2g
Carbohydrates: 8g
Net Carbohydrates: 6g
Sugar: 2g

GARLICKY GREEN BEANS

SERVES 2

At only 4.5 grams of net carbohydrates per cup, green beans are one of the only "beans" that fit into a keto lifestyle. When making this recipe, you can save yourself a bunch of prep time by buying a bag of green beans that have already been washed, cleaned, and trimmed for you.

½ pound green beans, trimmed

2 tablespoons grass-fed butter

1 clove garlic, minced

2 tablespoons toasted pine nuts

⅛ teaspoon salt

⅛ teaspoon black pepper

1 Bring a large pot of water to a boil. Add green beans and cook until fork tender, 4–5 minutes.

2 In a large skillet over medium heat, heat butter. Add garlic and pine nuts and sauté 3 minutes or until pine nuts are lightly browned.

3 Transfer green beans to skillet, add salt and pepper, and toss until coated. Serve hot.

PER SERVING
Calories: 190
Fat: 17g
Protein: 2g
Sodium: 414mg
Fiber: 2g
Carbohydrates: 6g
Net Carbohydrates: 4g
Sugar: 1g

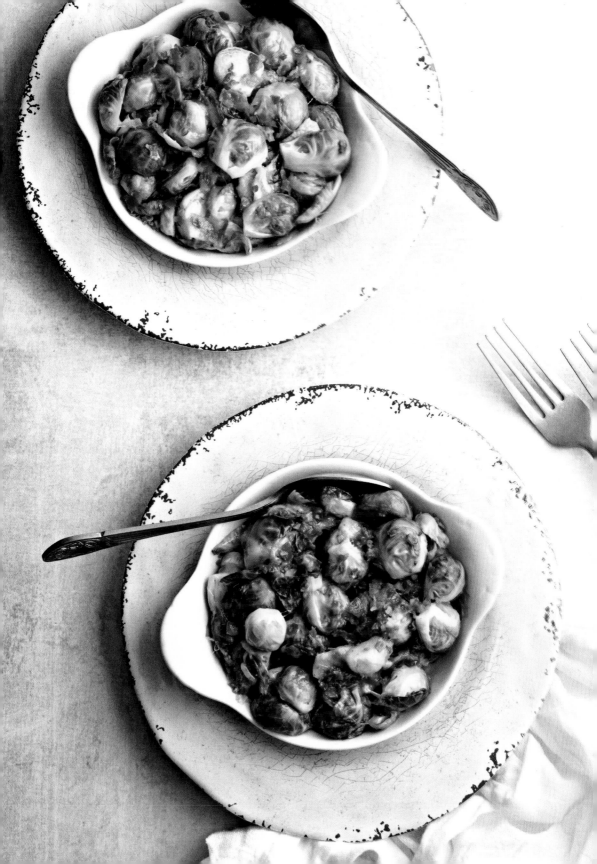

CHEESY BACON BRUSSELS SPROUTS

SERVES 2

Brussels sprouts may be one of the most scoffed at vegetables, but when you try them sautéed in bacon fat and with added cheese, they'll jump to the top of your list of favorites. After all, everything's better (especially on keto) with bacon, right?

3 slices no-sugar-added bacon

½ pound Brussels sprouts, trimmed and cut in half lengthwise

¾ cup shredded pepper jack cheese

PER SERVING
Calories: 369
Fat: 28g
Protein: 19g
Sodium: 552mg
Fiber: 3g
Carbohydrates: 8g
Net Carbohydrates: 5g
Sugar: 2g

1 In a large skillet over medium-high heat, cook bacon until crispy, about 10 minutes.

2 Remove bacon from pan and set aside. Add Brussels sprouts to hot pan and sauté until fork tender, about 8 minutes.

3 Chop bacon into small pieces and add to Brussels sprouts. Sprinkle cheese on top and stir until melted. Serve hot.

BENEFITS OF BRUSSELS SPROUTS

Serving for serving, Brussels sprouts contain significantly more vitamin C than an orange. They're also rich in vitamin A, beta-carotene, folic acid, iron, magnesium, selenium, and fiber. Chinese medicine practitioners also often recommend Brussels sprouts to help with digestive troubles, so if you're feeling constipated on keto, try adding them to your rotation.

CHAPTER 6

CHICKEN MAIN DISHES

Chicken is the go-to protein choice for most diet plans, and keto is no exception. It's lean, it's versatile, and it's easy to whip up when you don't know what else to make for dinner. But if you're eating chicken all the time, it's easy to fall into a monotony trap where you're making the same dishes day after day. This chapter uses chicken in everything from Zucchini Chicken Alfredo to a Chicken Cordon Bleu Casserole to Fried Chicken, with a keto-approved twist to keep those carbohydrates within range, of course.

If you're stuck in a chicken rut, you'll definitely find something to help snap you out of it. No boring chicken recipes here!

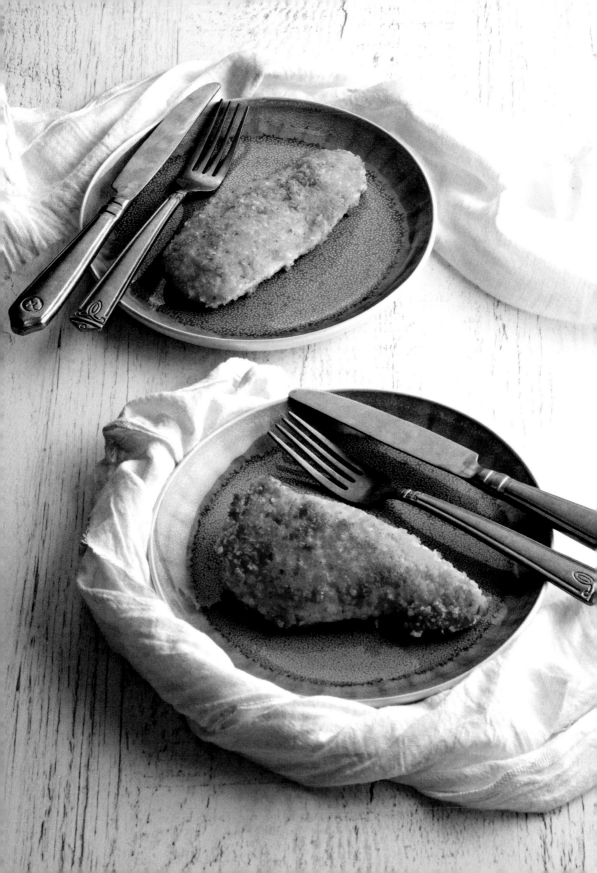

FRIED CHICKEN

SERVES 2

Who says you have to miss fried chicken when you're doing keto? If you want extra-crispy fried chicken, dip the chicken breasts in the pork rind mixture, then into the egg mixture, and then back into the pork rind mixture. This will create a thick coating and really crisp this Fried Chicken up.

½ cup crushed pork rinds

2 tablespoons grated Parmesan cheese

¼ teaspoon garlic powder

¼ teaspoon onion powder

¼ teaspoon dried minced onion

⅛ teaspoon salt

¼ teaspoon black pepper

1 large egg

2 (4-ounce) boneless, skinless chicken breasts

2 tablespoons coconut oil

PER SERVING

Calories: 356
Fat: 20g
Protein: 40g
Sodium: 474mg
Fiber: 0g
Carbohydrates: 1g
Net Carbohydrates: 1g
Sugar: 0g

1 Put pork rinds, Parmesan cheese, garlic powder, onion powder, minced onion, salt, and pepper in a large mixing bowl and stir until well combined.

2 Crack egg into a separate bowl and whisk.

3 Dip each chicken breast into egg and then coat in pork rind mixture, making sure the chicken is completely covered.

4 In a medium skillet over medium-high heat, heat coconut oil. When coconut oil is hot, place chicken breasts into pan. Let cook 5–7 minutes or until pork rind crust is browned. Flip chicken over and let cook another 5–7 minutes until cooked through.

5 Serve hot.

PICKING PORK RINDS

All pork rinds are not created equally. When choosing pork rinds, read the ingredient list and choose a package that comes from pigs that are humanely treated and contains only pork skin and pork fat or pork skin and salt. Avoid pork rinds with any added artificial ingredients that come from conventionally raised pigs.

ZUCCHINI CHICKEN ALFREDO

SERVES 2

This recipe calls for chicken, but shrimp makes a great substitute. If you use shrimp instead, you'll only add 1 gram of carbohydrate per 10 shrimp.

FOR ZUCCHINI CHICKEN

1 large zucchini

¼ teaspoon salt

¼ teaspoon black pepper

⅛ teaspoon paprika

⅛ teaspoon garlic powder

½ pound boneless, skinless chicken thighs

1 tablespoon coconut oil

1 tablespoon unsalted butter

FOR ALFREDO SAUCE

¼ cup unsalted butter

½ cup heavy cream

1½ tablespoons grated Asiago cheese

1½ tablespoons grated Parmesan cheese

¼ teaspoon granulated garlic

⅛ teaspoon ground nutmeg

⅛ teaspoon salt

⅛ teaspoon black pepper

PER SERVING

Calories: 695
Fat: 60g
Protein: 25g
Sodium: 644mg
Fiber: 2g
Carbohydrates: 8g
Net Carbohydrates: 6g
Sugar: 6g

1 Cut zucchini into long strips using vegetable peeler or spiralizer. Set aside on a paper towel and allow to sweat.

2 Sprinkle salt, pepper, paprika, and garlic powder over chicken thighs.

3 Heat coconut oil in a medium skillet over medium heat and place chicken in pan. Cook 5 minutes, flip over, and then cook another 5 minutes, or until no longer pink.

4 Remove chicken from heat with a slotted spoon and chop into large pieces.

5 Add butter to hot pan. Once butter melts, add zucchini and sauté until softened but still firm, about 5 minutes.

6 To make sauce: In a medium saucepan over medium heat, melt butter. Add heavy cream and whisk 2 minutes. Add Asiago cheese and Parmesan cheese and whisk until melted. Continue to cook about 5 minutes, allowing mixture to simmer.

7 Stir in garlic, nutmeg, salt, and pepper. Remove from heat.

8 To assemble: Add Alfredo sauce and chopped chicken to pan with zucchini and toss until coated.

STOCKING UP ON CHICKEN

Chicken thighs are regularly on sale because they are less popular than chicken breasts. Take advantage of these sales by buying several packages at a time and freezing them for later. You can even cook the chicken before freezing to save time when making recipes down the road.

SPICY CHICKEN AND AVOCADO CASSEROLE

SERVES 2

You can replace the chicken in this recipe with canned tuna, ground beef or pork, or diced chunks of ham for different variations on protein that don't change the carbohydrate count much. Serve it for dinner or split it in two and package it up for lunch.

1 medium avocado, peeled, pitted, and roughly chopped

1 tablespoon coconut oil

¼ cup diced yellow onion

½ cup diced green bell pepper

1 (12.5-ounce) can shredded chicken breast

3 tablespoons sour cream

3 tablespoons keto-friendly mayonnaise

½ cup shredded Cheddar cheese, divided

1/16 teaspoon red pepper flakes

⅛ teaspoon salt

⅛ teaspoon black pepper

PER SERVING
Calories: 775
Fat: 57g
Protein: 49g
Sodium: 1,206mg
Fiber: 6g
Carbohydrates: 12g
Net Carbohydrates: 6g
Sugar: 3g

1 Preheat oven to 350°F.

2 Spread chopped avocados along the bottom of a 9" × 5" baking pan.

3 In a medium skillet over medium-high heat, heat coconut oil. Add onions and cook until lightly browned, about 3 minutes. Add bell pepper and cook until soft, another 3 minutes. Remove from heat.

4 In a medium mixing bowl, place chicken, sour cream, mayonnaise, ¼ cup Cheddar cheese, red pepper flakes, salt, and black pepper and stir until combined. Add onions and bell peppers.

5 Spoon mixture over avocados. Top with remaining ¼ cup Cheddar cheese.

6 Bake 20 minutes or until cheese is slightly browned and casserole is bubbling.

7 Allow to cool slightly before serving.

GO CRAZY FOR COCONUT OIL

Coconut oil is a staple on the ketogenic diet. The oil is resistant to high heat, so unlike olive oil, it doesn't oxidize with high temperatures. Coconut oil also contains medium-chain triglycerides, a type of fat that provides your body with immediate energy and can help boost metabolism.

STUFFED CHICKEN BREAST

SERVES 2

When using frozen spinach, make sure it's completely thawed and drained before using it. If there's excess water, squeeze it dry with your hands or a cheesecloth before adding it to the filling. If you don't, your Stuffed Chicken Breast may come out a little runny.

2 (4-ounce) boneless, skinless chicken breasts

1 ounce cream cheese, softened

2 tablespoons sour cream

½ (10-ounce) package fresh spinach, chopped

2 tablespoons chopped fresh basil

1½ teaspoons minced green onions

¼ cup shredded pepper jack cheese

1 clove garlic, minced

¼ teaspoon salt

¼ teaspoon black pepper

1 Preheat oven to 375°F.

2 Cut a slit into the side of each chicken breast to create a pocket.

3 Combine all other ingredients in a medium bowl and beat until smooth.

4 Fill each chicken breast with half of mixture and secure pocket closed with toothpicks.

5 Place chicken breasts in a baking pan and cook 35 minutes, or until chicken is no longer pink.

PER SERVING
Calories: 266
Fat: 13g
Protein: 32g
Sodium: 529mg
Fiber: 2g
Carbohydrates: 5g
Net Carbohydrates: 3g
Sugar: 1g

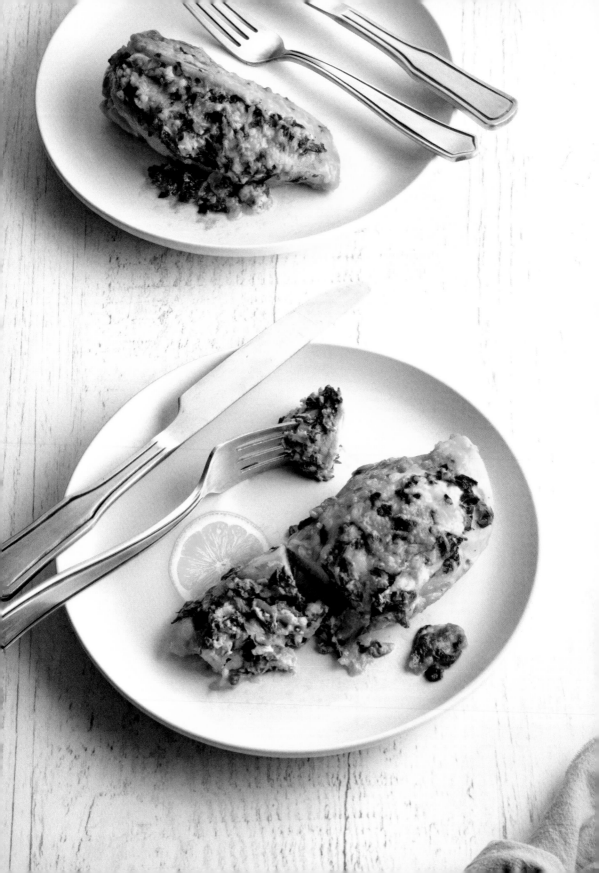

TURKEY AVOCADO ROLLS

SERVES 2

Lemon pepper has a strong taste, so in this recipe, a little goes a long way. Try the recipe as written before deciding if you need more. If you don't like the zing of lemon, try garlic pepper in place of the lemon pepper or just omit the spice blend completely.

6 (1-ounce) slices turkey breast

6 (1-ounce) slices Swiss cheese

1½ cups baby spinach

½ large avocado, peeled, pitted, and cut into 6 slices

2 tablespoons keto-friendly mayonnaise

⅛ teaspoon lemon pepper

1 Lay out slices of turkey breast flat and place one slice Swiss cheese on top of each one.

2 Top each slice with ¼ cup baby spinach and one slice avocado. Drizzle with 1 teaspoon mayonnaise.

3 Sprinkle each "sandwich" with lemon pepper. Roll up sandwiches and secure with toothpicks. Serve immediately or refrigerate until ready to serve.

PER SERVING

Calories: 631
Fat: 44g
Protein: 48g
Sodium: 250mg
Fiber: 3g
Carbohydrates: 8g
Net Carbohydrates: 5g
Sugar: 1g

CHECK YOUR SPICES

It may come as a surprise, but many commercial spices contain sugar or hydrogenated fats. Don't assume that an ingredient, such as lemon pepper, is free of carbohydrates until you check the label. If it contains sugar, ditch it and find one that doesn't. When it comes to herbs and spices, there are plenty of sugar-free options out there.

CHICKEN CORDON BLEU CASSEROLE

SERVES 2

Traditional chicken cordon bleu contains a combination of ham, chicken, and Swiss cheese, but if you're not a fan of the bite of Swiss cheese, swap it out for a cheese with a milder flavor, such as provolone or mozzarella.

1 cup cooked chopped chicken breast

½ cup cooked diced sugar-free ham

½ cup cubed Swiss cheese

¼ cup heavy cream

¼ cup sour cream

2 ounces cream cheese

¼ teaspoon granulated garlic

¼ teaspoon granulated onion

⅛ teaspoon salt

⅛ teaspoon black pepper

¼ cup crushed pork rinds

1 Preheat oven to 350°F.

2 Mix chicken and ham and spread out in the bottom of a 9" × 5" baking pan. Sprinkle Swiss cheese on top of chicken and ham.

3 In a medium saucepan over medium heat, heat heavy cream, sour cream, and cream cheese until cream cheese is melted and mixture is smooth. Add garlic, onion, salt, and pepper. Pour mixture over chicken, ham, and Swiss cheese.

4 Sprinkle pork rinds across top of casserole. Bake 30 minutes, or until slightly browned and cheese is bubbly.

PER SERVING
Calories: 556
Fat: 37g
Protein: 41g
Sodium: 834mg
Fiber: 0g
Carbohydrates: 5g
Net Carbohydrates: 5g
Sugar: 3g

BACON-WRAPPED CHICKEN

SERVES 2

If you want to make sure your bacon comes out really crispy, you can partially cook the bacon in a skillet before wrapping it around the chicken. This will help ensure that the bacon is thoroughly cooked by the time the chicken comes out of the oven.

2 (4-ounce) boneless, skinless chicken breasts

4 ounces cream cheese, softened

¼ cup shredded pepper jack cheese

1 tablespoon dried chives

⅛ teaspoon salt

⅛ teaspoon black pepper

2 slices no-sugar-added bacon

PER SERVING
Calories: 422
Fat: 27g
Protein: 36g
Sodium: 671mg
Fiber: 0g
Carbohydrates: 3g
Net Carbohydrates: 3g
Sugar: 2g

1 Preheat oven to 400°F.

2 Cut a pocket into each chicken breast with a small paring knife. Set aside.

3 In a medium bowl, combine cream cheese, pepper jack cheese, chives, salt, and pepper and mix until combined.

4 Fill each chicken breast with half of cream cheese mixture and wrap with one bacon slice. Secure with a toothpick.

5 Place chicken breasts in a baking pan and bake 35 minutes or until a meat thermometer reads 165°F.

6 Turn oven to broil and broil on top rack until bacon is crispy, about 5 minutes.

CHICKEN AND AVOCADO SALAD

SERVES 2

Precooked canned chicken makes this recipe a cinch to whip up, but if you have extra time, you can cook some boneless, skinless chicken breasts (or some chicken thighs if you want more fat), shred them or cut them into cubes, and use that instead.

1 (12.5-ounce) can shredded chicken breast

1 medium avocado, peeled, pitted, and cubed

¼ cup keto-friendly mayonnaise

2 tablespoons sliced black olives

¼ teaspoon garlic salt

¼ teaspoon black pepper

⅛ teaspoon paprika

1 teaspoon fresh lemon juice

1 teaspoon olive oil

Put all ingredients in a medium mixing bowl and mash with a fork until combined.

PER SERVING

Calories: 638

Fat: 49g

Protein: 41g

Sodium: 1,218mg

Fiber: 5g

Carbohydrates: 8g

Net Carbohydrates: 3g

Sugar: 0g

SPINACH, FETA, AND APPLE SALAD

SERVES 2

Granny Smith apples tend to be lower in sugar than sweeter varieties. If you have some carbohydrates to spare and want a bit of a sweeter taste, swap the Granny Smith apple for another apple of your choice. Serve this salad with Tessemae's Green Goddess dressing.

4 cups baby spinach

8 ounces cooked chicken, cubed

½ cup chopped red onion

½ cup crumbled feta cheese

½ small Granny Smith apple, diced

½ cup toasted pine nuts

Combine all ingredients in a medium bowl and toss to coat. Serve immediately.

PER SERVING

Calories: 572

Fat: 32g

Protein: 47g

Sodium: 479mg

Fiber: 4g

Carbohydrates: 17g

Net Carbohydrates: 13g

Sugar: 8g

THE CARBS IN APPLES

A small Granny Smith apple contains 21 grams of carbohydrates, almost 4 grams of which come from fiber. Because one apple's net carbohydrate count is 17 grams, you have to make sure you only eat them in moderation when following a keto diet.

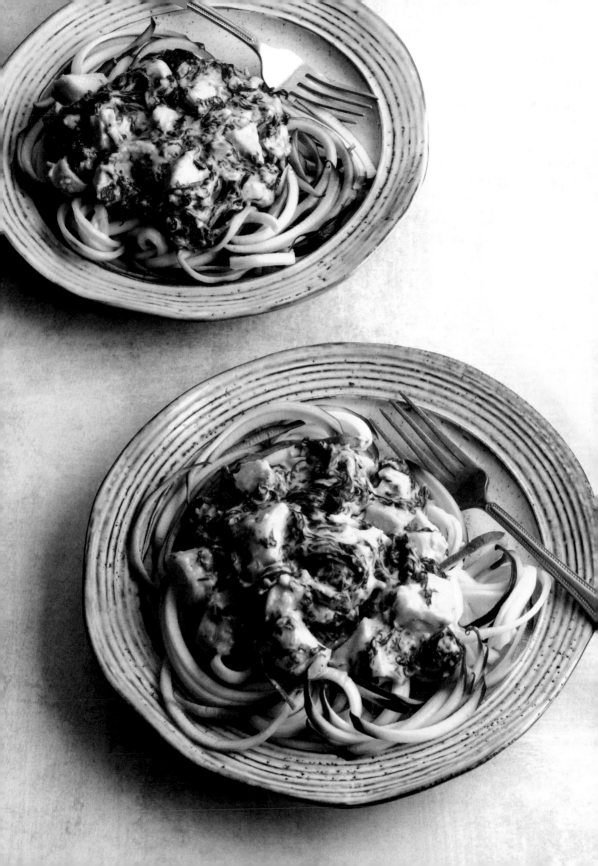

CREAMY CHICKEN ZOODLES

SERVES 2

This recipe calls for zucchini noodles, or "zoodles," which you can easily make with a vegetable spiralizer. You can find a spiralizer at most home stores, but if you prefer, you can also make zucchini noodles by julienning the zucchini with a vegetable peeler.

1 large zucchini

1 tablespoon extra-virgin olive oil

½ pound boneless, skinless chicken breasts, cut into cubes

¼ teaspoon salt

¼ teaspoon black pepper

2½ cups fresh spinach

3 ounces cream cheese

1 tablespoon grated Parmesan cheese

1 tablespoon feta cheese crumbles

PER SERVING

Calories: 386
Fat: 23g
Protein: 32g
Sodium: 617mg
Fiber: 3g
Carbohydrates: 9g
Net Carbohydrates: 6g
Sugar: 6g

1 Cut zucchini in long strips with a vegetable peeler or a spiralizer. Set zucchini aside on a paper towel and allow to sweat.

2 In a medium skillet over medium heat, heat olive oil. Season chicken cubes with salt and pepper and add to hot pan. Cook chicken until no longer pink, about 10 minutes.

3 Remove chicken from pan with a slotted spoon and set aside.

4 Add spinach to hot pan and sauté until wilted. Add cream cheese, Parmesan cheese, and feta cheese, and stir until melted.

5 Add chicken back to pan and toss until coated. Remove from heat and pour over zucchini noodles.

CHAPTER 7

PORK MAIN DISHES

Although chicken is the go-to protein source for many different diets, pork has earned its rightful place on the keto diet. Unlike other plans, which require you to swap out fattier cuts of meat, like pork, for leaner varieties, keto embraces the higher fat content of pork. You can eat ham and bacon as well as pork chops and pork tenderloin. No cut is off-limits.

However, if you're including things like bacon and sausage, make sure to read your labels and double-check that there's no added sugar and that the brands you're choosing have as few added ingredients as possible.

Once you've chosen your high-quality ingredients, you can incorporate them into all of the two-serving, mouth-watering recipes—like Ham and Cheese Casserole, Breadless BLT, and Stuffed Pork Tenderloin—that you'll find in this chapter.

HAM AND CHEESE CASSEROLE

SERVES 2

Don't forget to allow the cream cheese to reach room temperature before starting this recipe. Softened cream cheese is much easier to work with than cream cheese fresh from the refrigerator, especially when you're mixing it with other ingredients. If you're short on time, you can put the cream cheese in the microwave for a few seconds to soften it quickly.

2 cups cauliflower florets

2 ounces cream cheese, softened

3 tablespoons heavy cream

¾ cup cooked cubed no-sugar-added ham

⅓ cup shredded Cheddar cheese

2 teaspoons grated Parmesan cheese

1 tablespoon chopped green onion

¼ teaspoon salt

¼ teaspoon black pepper

1 Preheat oven to 350°F.

2 Bring a large pot of water to a boil and add cauliflower. Boil until cauliflower is fork tender, about 5–10 minutes. Strain cauliflower and return to pot.

3 Put cream cheese and heavy cream in a medium mixing bowl and beat with a handheld beater until smooth. Transfer cream cheese mixture to cauliflower in pot and stir until cauliflower is coated. Add in ham, Cheddar cheese, Parmesan cheese, green onions, salt, and pepper and stir until combined.

4 Transfer mixture to a 9" × 5" baking pan and bake until cheese is melted and casserole is bubbly, about 30 minutes. Serve hot.

PER SERVING

Calories: 372
Fat: 26g
Protein: 21g
Sodium: 1,319mg
Fiber: 2g
Carbohydrates: 8g
Net Carbohydrates: 6g
Sugar: 4g

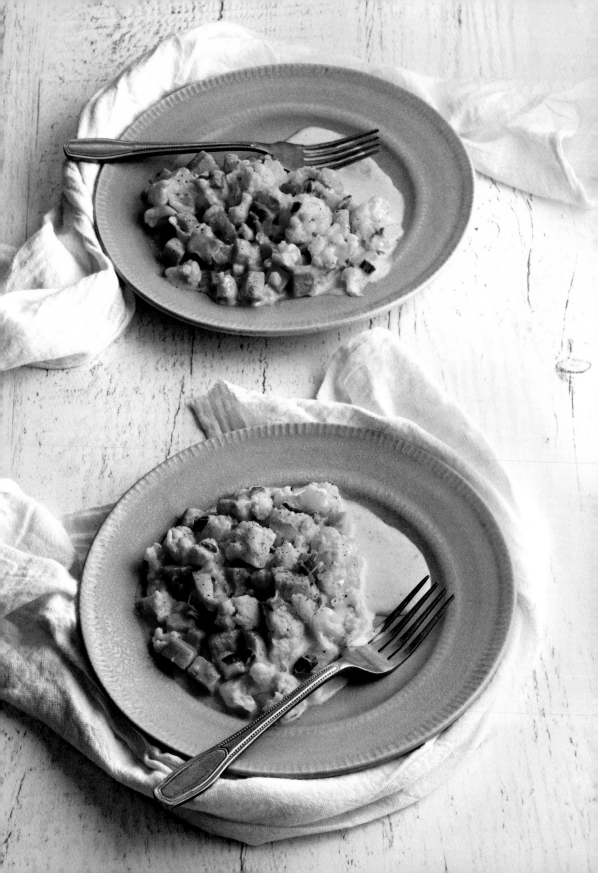

PEPPERONI PIZZA CASSEROLE

SERVES 2

Instead of pepperoni, you can use salami or prosciutto in this recipe. Just read the ingredients and make sure that the cured meats don't contain any added sugar. You can also add any of your favorite keto-friendly pizza toppings to satisfy your pizza cravings.

2 cups cauliflower florets

1 tablespoon grass-fed butter

2 tablespoons heavy cream

2 teaspoons grated Parmesan cheese

½ teaspoon Italian seasoning

⅓ cup mozzarella cheese, divided

¼ cup no-sugar-added pizza sauce

6 slices sugar-free pepperoni

PER SERVING
Calories: 246
Fat: 19g
Protein: 9g
Sodium: 423mg
Fiber: 3g
Carbohydrates: 10g
Net Carbohydrates: 7g
Sugar: 3g

1 Preheat oven to 375°F.

2 Bring a large pot of water to a boil and add cauliflower florets. Boil until fork tender, about 5–7 minutes.

3 Strain cauliflower and put into a food processor or blender. While cauliflower is still hot, add butter and heavy cream, and process or blend until smooth. Add Parmesan cheese, Italian seasoning, and 2 tablespoons mozzarella cheese and process until smooth.

4 Pour cauliflower mixture into a 9" × 5" pan and spread it out evenly. Pour pizza sauce over cauliflower mixture.

5 Top with remaining mozzarella cheese and pepperoni. Bake 20 minutes or until cheese is slightly browned and casserole is bubbling.

CREAMY ROSEMARY AND PROSCIUTTO-BAKED AVOCADOS

SERVES 2

This recipe sounds fancy, but names can be deceiving, so don't let that scare you away. These Creamy Rosemary and Prosciutto–Baked Avocados are easy to make, calling for only a handful of ingredients, and can be ready in a matter of minutes.

2 medium avocados, halved and pitted, skin on

2 ounces cream cheese

1 tablespoon finely chopped fresh rosemary

2 ounces cooked prosciutto, crumbled

1 Preheat oven to 350°F.

2 Place avocado halves, hole side up, in a shallow ramekin or ovenproof dish just large enough to hold them.

3 In a small bowl, mix cream cheese with rosemary and prosciutto.

4 Place half of mixture into each avocado cavity.

5 Bake 20 minutes. Serve hot.

PER SERVING

Calories: 407
Fat: 33g
Protein: 10g
Sodium: 226mg
Fiber: 9g
Carbohydrates: 14g
Net Carbohydrates: 5g
Sugar: 1g

PORTOBELLO PIZZAS

SERVES 2

These Portobello Pizzas call for pepperoni and cheese, one of the most basic pizza combinations, but you can use whatever keto-approved toppings that you like. Try sausage and green bell peppers or prosciutto and mushrooms or pepperoni and feta cheese. You can even make one to your liking and one tailored to your eating partner's preferences. The possibilities are endless!

2 large portobello mushrooms

2 teaspoons olive oil

½ cup no-sugar-added marinara sauce

½ cup shredded mozzarella cheese

6 slices no-sugar-added pepperoni

PER SERVING

Calories: 192
Fat: 13g
Protein: 11g
Sodium: 423mg
Fiber: 2g
Carbohydrates: 9g
Net Carbohydrates: 7g
Sugar: 5g

1 Preheat oven to 375°F.

2 Remove stems from mushrooms and brush each cap inside and outside with 1 teaspoon olive oil. Place on a foil-lined baking sheet and bake stem side down for 10 minutes.

3 Remove mushrooms from oven and fill each cap with ¼ cup marinara sauce, ¼ cup mozzarella cheese, and three slices pepperoni.

4 Return to oven and cook another 10 minutes or until cheese is lightly browned and bubbly. Serve hot.

DELI ROLLUPS

SERVES 2

Instead of purchasing prepared chive cream cheese, which often contains added ingredients that you might not want on your keto plan, you can make your own by combining a plain high-quality cream cheese with minced dried onions and dried chives.

8 (1-ounce) slices sugar-free deli ham

½ cup chive cream cheese

1 cup chopped baby spinach

1 medium red bell pepper, seeded and sliced

PER SERVING
Calories: 340
Fat: 21g
Protein: 23g
Sodium: 1,267mg
Fiber: 2g
Carbohydrates: 9g
Net Carbohydrates: 7g
Sugar: 6g

1 Lay out each slice of ham flat. Take 1 tablespoon cream cheese and spread it on a slice of ham. Repeat for the remaining slices.

2 Put 2 tablespoons chopped spinach on top of the cream cheese on each slice.

3 Divide bell pepper into eight equal portions and put each portion on top of spinach.

4 Roll up the ham and secure with a toothpick. Eat immediately or refrigerate until ready to serve.

CHECK YOUR LABELS!

Many hams contain cane sugar, brown sugar, maple syrup, or honey. When choosing a ham, read your labels carefully and stay away from any that contain added sugars, which will up the carbohydrate content of this meal significantly. If you can't find ham without added sugar, you can use prosciutto instead.

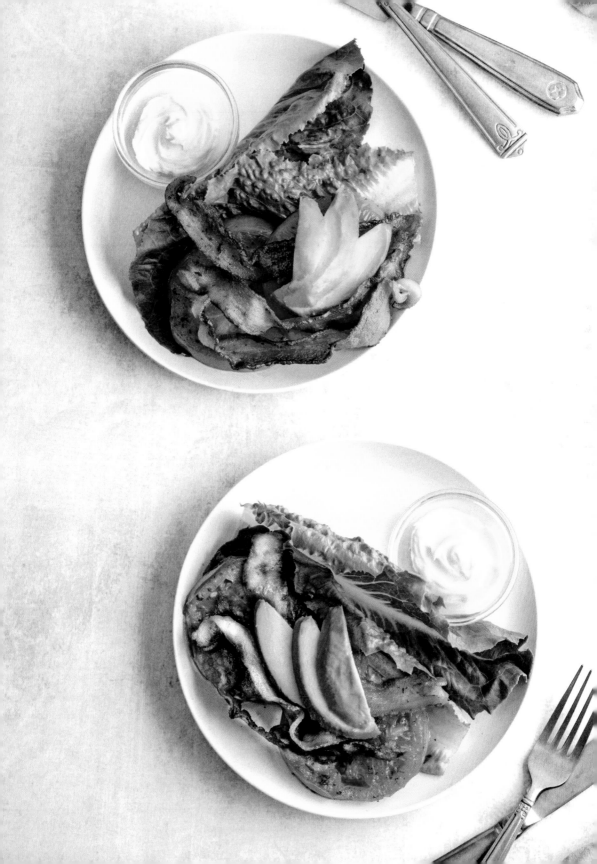

BREADLESS BLT

SERVES 2

When cooking the tomato for this recipe, you just want to char it slightly to add some extra flavor, but you want to try not to cook it through completely. If the tomato gets too soft, it won't hold up as well.

6 slices sugar-free bacon

1 large tomato, cut into 4 equal slices

4 leaves romaine lettuce

½ large avocado, peeled, pitted, and sliced

2 tablespoons olive oil mayonnaise

1 In a medium skillet over medium heat, cook bacon until crisp. Remove bacon and return bacon fat to heat.

2 Place each tomato slice in bacon fat and cook 1 minute. Remove from pan and set aside.

3 Place one piece of romaine lettuce on each plate and top each with two tomato slices, three strips bacon, half of the avocado slices, and 1 tablespoon mayonnaise.

4 Cover with remaining romaine leaves and serve.

PER SERVING

Calories: 293
Fat: 21g
Protein: 14g
Sodium: 696mg
Fiber: 5g
Carbohydrates: 10g
Net Carbohydrates: 5g
Sugar: 3g

GROUND PORK STIR-FRY

SERVES 2

You can change the flavor profile of this recipe by simply changing the spices you use. Use rosemary and thyme instead of garlic, onion, and sage or go for a smoked flavor with a little bit of spice by using paprika and chili powder. Changing the spices is an easy way to add variation to prevent boredom on your keto plan.

1 tablespoon coconut oil

½ medium yellow onion, peeled and sliced

2 cloves garlic, minced

1 small zucchini, diced

½ pound ground pork

½ (10-ounce) bag fresh spinach

½ cup chopped cooked broccoli

½ teaspoon ground sage

½ teaspoon granulated garlic

½ teaspoon granulated onion

½ teaspoon salt

½ teaspoon black pepper

¼ teaspoon red pepper flakes

1 small avocado, peeled, pitted, and diced

PER SERVING
Calories: 479
Fat: 32g
Protein: 26g
Sodium: 740mg
Fiber: 9g
Carbohydrates: 19g
Net Carbohydrates: 10g
Sugar: 4g

1 In a medium skillet over medium-high heat, heat coconut oil. Add sliced onion and minced garlic and sauté until transparent, about 5 minutes.

2 Add zucchini and sauté until soft, another 3–4 minutes. Add ground pork and sauté until no longer pink.

3 When meat is cooked, add spinach and sauté until wilted. Add broccoli, sage, granulated garlic, granulated onion, salt, pepper, and red pepper flakes. Toss mixture until evenly covered with spices.

4 Remove from heat and divide into two bowls. Top each serving with half of avocado.

MAKE AHEAD FOR MAXIMUM FLAVOR

Many stir-fry recipes taste even better after they sit overnight since the flavors have more time to meld together and develop. If you want to prepare it in advance, follow the instructions and then transfer to a glass airtight container. When it's time to eat, heat it up over low heat on the stove. When you serve stir-fry, you can even put a fried egg on top to increase the fat and protein content.

SPINACH AND PROSCIUTTO SALAD

SERVES 2

The unsalted cashews in this recipe help satisfy that craving for something crunchy when you're eating a salad. As a bonus, they taste great with avocado, but watch your portions because they are a higher-carb nut. Serve this Spinach and Prosciutto Salad with Tessemae's Balsamic Vinaigrette or Green Goddess dressing (the nutrition stats for this recipe are for the salad only, and don't include the stats for whatever salad dressing you use).

4 cups baby spinach

6 ounces prosciutto

1 large avocado, peeled, pitted, and diced

¼ cup diced red onion

¼ cup chopped raw unsalted cashews

PER SERVING
Calories: 488
Fat: 36g
Protein: 25g
Sodium: 394mg
Fiber: 7g
Carbohydrates: 18g
Net Carbohydrates: 11g
Sugar: 2g

1 Put spinach in a large mixing bowl. Dice prosciutto and put on top of spinach. Put avocado, red onion, and cashews on top of spinach.

2 Add keto dressing of your choice to salad and toss to coat. Serve immediately.

BE CHOOSY WITH NUTS

When buying nuts, opt for raw, unsalted varieties rather than roasted, salted, or sugared versions. Raw nuts generally contain no added ingredients, while roasted, flavored nuts can contain unhealthy oils and sugar. Aside from being unhealthy, these added ingredients can add a considerable amount of carbs.

STUFFED PORK TENDERLOIN

SERVES 2

Pork tenderloin is so versatile that you can eat this recipe as is or use it as a basic template and change the fillings to any keto-approved options you want. Try ham instead of prosciutto or Gorgonzola cheese or blue cheese instead of feta.

½ pound pork tenderloin

2 (0.5-ounce) slices prosciutto

2 slices no-sugar-added bacon, cooked and chopped

¼ teaspoon garlic powder

¼ teaspoon ground sage

¼ teaspoon black pepper

⅛ teaspoon salt

¼ teaspoon dry mustard

2 ounces cream cheese, softened

2 tablespoons feta cheese crumbles

½ cup frozen spinach, thawed

1½ tablespoons extra-virgin olive oil

PER SERVING

Calories: 431
Fat: 30g
Protein: 31g
Sodium: 812mg
Fiber: 1g
Carbohydrates: 5g
Net Carbohydrates: 4g
Sugar: 2g

1 Preheat oven to 350°F.

2 Butterfly pork tenderloin. Lay each slice of prosciutto down on the pork.

3 In a medium mixing bowl, put bacon, garlic powder, spices, cream cheese, feta cheese, and spinach and beat until smooth.

4 Spread filling over prosciutto and roll tenderloin closed. Secure pork with a kitchen string.

5 In a large pan over medium-high heat, heat olive oil. Sear pork 2 minutes on each side, then place in a baking pan.

6 Bake 30 minutes or until inside is no longer pink and thermometer reads 160°F.

PROSCIUTTO VERSUS BACON

Prosciutto and bacon are both made from pork, but the two cured meats do have characteristics that separate them from each other. Bacon is cured and then smoked using a cold-smoking process. Because the smoking temperature is low, the bacon never gets heated and stays raw. On the other hand, prosciutto is cured but not smoked. Like bacon, it stays raw, but doesn't have the same smoky flavor.

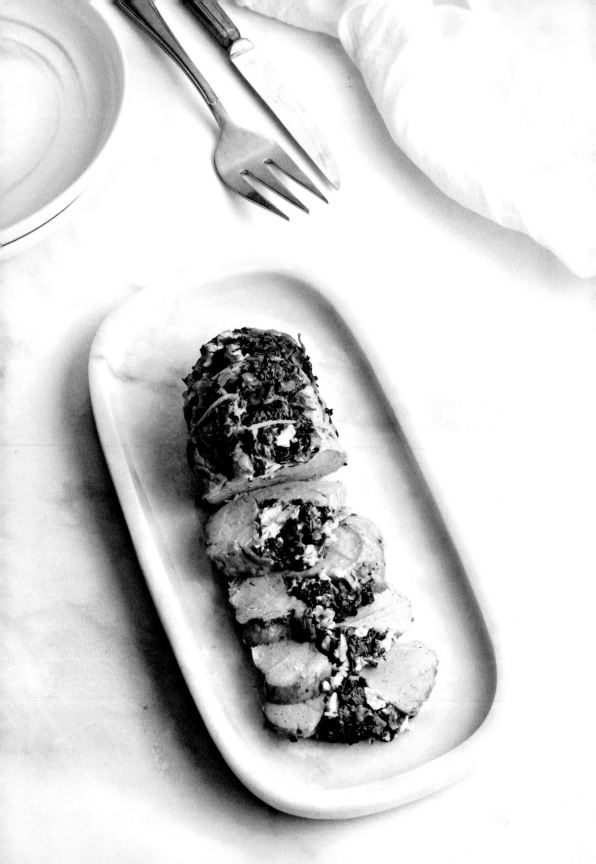

CHAPTER 8

BEEF MAIN DISHES

There's a reason beef is the second most popular meat choice in America, with each person eating an average of 54 pounds of the red meat every year. It's versatile, it's easy to cook, and, of course, it's delicious. If you're cooking with ground beef, you can also choose different fat contents to fit into your macros. If you have room for more fat, use an 80/20 beef. If you want to go a little leaner, opt for a 90/10. The choice is yours.

This chapter uses different forms of beef in everything from Roast Beef Lettuce Wraps to Taco Bowls to "Spaghetti" and Spicy Meatballs. Whatever recipe you choose, it's sure to satisfy the both of you.

KETO MEATLOAF

SERVES 2

Who says you need bread crumbs to hold a meatloaf together? This keto-friendly recipe uses an egg as a binder instead, which keeps the carbohydrate count low while also increasing the content of fat, protein, and various vitamins and minerals in the finished dish.

1 tablespoon grass-fed salted butter

1 small yellow onion, peeled and diced

2 cloves garlic, minced

2 slices no-sugar-added bacon, cooked

½ pound 85/15 lean ground beef

1 large egg

½ teaspoon dried thyme

½ teaspoon dried parsley

¼ teaspoon dry mustard

¼ teaspoon salt

⅛ teaspoon black pepper

PER SERVING
Calories: 406
Fat: 26g
Protein: 29g
Sodium: 613mg
Fiber: 1g
Carbohydrates: 5g
Net Carbohydrates: 4g
Sugar: 2g

1 Preheat oven to 350°F.

2 In a large skillet over medium-high heat, heat butter until melted. Add onions and garlic and sauté until softened, 3–4 minutes. Remove from heat and set aside to cool.

3 Chop bacon and put in a large mixing bowl. Add ground beef, egg, herbs, spices, and garlic and onion mixture and mix until evenly incorporated.

4 Transfer meat mixture to a mini loaf pan, evenly dividing the meat between two of the cavities in the pan.

5 Cook 50 minutes or until a meat thermometer inserted in the center reads 165°F. Let the loaves rest 10 minutes before serving.

THE EGG-CELLENT EGG

Eggs were shunned in the low-fat era of the 1990s, but as most keto dieters now know, the fear was unwarranted. Eggs are one of the most nutritious foods out there. In addition to the fact that they don't contain any carbohydrates, they also contain almost every vitamin and mineral, with the exception of vitamin C. They're also rich in protein and choline, a compound found in the yolk that helps keep your liver healthy and allows your body to access all the nutrients it needs.

COTTAGE PIE

SERVES 2

This Cottage Pie is a great way to use up any leftover vegetables that you have in your refrigerator at the end of the week. Although the recipe calls for cauliflower and onion, you can add any low-carbohydrate options that you both like. Zucchini, summer squash, and broccoli are all great options.

1 tablespoon coconut oil

¼ cup chopped yellow onion

1 clove garlic, minced

1 medium stalk celery, diced

½ cup diced zucchini

½ pound 80/20 ground beef

½ teaspoon dried rosemary

¼ teaspoon dried thyme

¼ teaspoon black pepper

¼ teaspoon table salt

¼ teaspoon garlic powder

1 cup cauliflower florets, boiled

2 tablespoons heavy cream

1 tablespoon grass-fed butter

¼ teaspoon garlic salt

¼ cup shredded Cheddar cheese

1 Preheat oven to 350°F.

2 In a large skillet over medium-high heat, heat coconut oil. When oil is hot, add onions and garlic and sauté until translucent, about 5 minutes. Add celery and zucchini and sauté until soft, another 5 minutes.

3 Add beef, herbs, spices, and garlic powder and cook until no longer pink. Pour beef mixture into a 9" × 5" baking pan.

4 Put boiled cauliflower, heavy cream, butter, and garlic salt in a food processor and process until smooth. Pour cauliflower mixture on top of beef. Top with cheese.

5 Bake until cheese is melted and pie is bubbly, about 25 minutes. Allow to cool 10 minutes before serving.

PER SERVING

Calories: 508
Fat: 38g
Protein: 25g
Sodium: 754mg
Fiber: 2g
Carbohydrates: 8g
Net Carbohydrates: 6g
Sugar: 3g

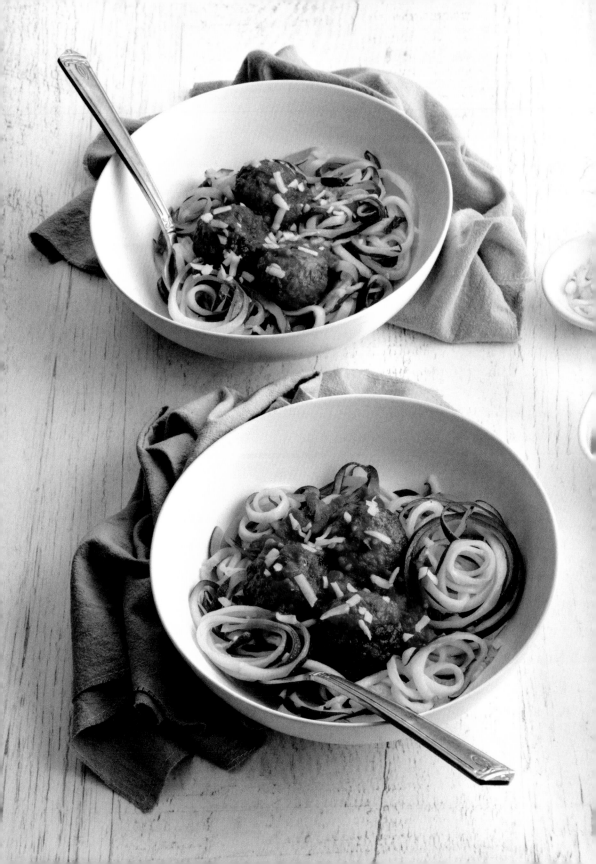

"SPAGHETTI" AND SPICY MEATBALLS

SERVES 2

When you taste this recipe, you won't even miss regular pasta noodles. The zucchini noodles have a mild flavor that serves as the perfect vehicle for the sauce and meatballs, which is the most important part of any "pasta" dish anyway, right?

1 large zucchini

1 tablespoon extra-virgin olive oil

½ cup chopped white onion

1 clove garlic, minced

1 large egg

⅛ cup shredded pepper jack cheese

¼ teaspoon salt

⅛ teaspoon black pepper

¼ pound 85/15 ground beef

¼ pound ground pork

1 tablespoon grass-fed salted butter

1 cup no-sugar-added marinara sauce

1 Preheat oven to 375°F.

2 Cut zucchini into long strips using a vegetable slicer or a spiralizer. Set aside onto a paper towel and allow to sweat.

3 In a large skillet over medium-high heat, heat olive oil. Add onions and garlic and sauté until transparent, 3–4 minutes. Set aside and allow to cool.

4 In a large mixing bowl, put egg, cheese, salt, pepper, beef, and pork. Add onion and garlic mixture and mix until evenly incorporated.

5 Shape meat mixture into six meatballs. Place meatballs on a baking sheet and bake 20 minutes or until internal temperature reaches 165°F.

6 In a large skillet over medium heat, heat butter. Add zucchini noodles and sauté, stirring frequently, until softened but still firm, about 5 minutes. Remove from heat.

7 Divide zucchini up into two servings. Top each serving with three meatballs and ½ cup marinara sauce.

PER SERVING

Calories: 363
Fat: 22g
Protein: 20g
Sodium: 744mg
Fiber: 4g
Carbohydrates: 20g
Net Carbohydrates: 16g
Sugar: 12g

ROAST BEEF LETTUCE WRAPS

SERVES 2

These lettuce wraps are incredibly easy to take with you on the go. When you're in a rush or have a busy day, you prepare a few in the morning and pack them away for both of your lunches later in the day.

4 (1-ounce) slices rare roast beef

4 large iceberg lettuce leaves

2 tablespoons keto-friendly mayonnaise

4 (1-ounce) slices provolone cheese

½ cup baby spinach

1 Place 1 slice roast beef in each lettuce wrap.

2 Spread ½ tablespoon mayonnaise on each piece of roast beef.

3 Top mayonnaise with 1 slice provolone cheese and ⅛ cup baby spinach.

4 Roll lettuce up around toppings. Serve immediately.

PER SERVING

Calories: 400
Fat: 30g
Protein: 31g
Sodium: 612mg

Fiber: 1g
Carbohydrates: 2g
Net Carbohydrates: 1g
Sugar: 1g

TACO BOWLS

SERVES 2

If you prefer to mimic more traditional tacos instead of putting all of your ingredients into a bowl, you can place the filling for these Taco Bowls into large leaves of iceberg lettuce and fold them up like tacos. It's the perfect Taco Tuesday date night recipe for two.

½ pound 85/15 lean ground beef

1 tablespoon taco seasoning

1 small avocado, peeled, pitted, and chopped

½ cup shredded Cheddar cheese

½ cup sour cream

¼ cup sliced black olives

1 In a large skillet over medium heat, brown ground beef. Without draining fat, add taco seasoning and stir until liquid is absorbed and beef is covered with seasoning.

2 Divide the beef between two bowls. Top beef in each bowl with half of avocado, ¼ cup cheese, ¼ cup sour cream, and ⅛ cup olives.

PER SERVING

Calories: 625
Fat: 45g
Protein: 31g
Sodium: 725mg

Fiber: 5g
Carbohydrates: 11g
Net Carbohydrates: 6g
Sugar: 2g

PEPPERONI MEAT-ZA

SERVES 2

Following a ketogenic diet doesn't mean that you have to give up pizza for good. If it did, no one would want to follow it, right? For this Pepperoni Meat-Za, you simply swap out the carbohydrate-filled crust for a crust made of meat and you're good to go.

½ pound 85/15 ground beef

1 large egg

¼ teaspoon garlic powder

¼ teaspoon onion powder

¼ teaspoon salt

¼ teaspoon black pepper

½ teaspoon dried oregano

2 tablespoons grated Parmesan cheese

¾ cup no-sugar-added marinara sauce

¾ cup shredded mozzarella cheese

8 slices sugar-free pepperoni

1 Preheat oven to 400°F.

2 In a large mixing bowl, mix meat and egg together until combined. Add garlic powder, onion powder, salt, pepper, oregano, and Parmesan cheese and mix. Press meat mixture into a 5" pie plate, forming a pizza crust.

3 Bake 20 minutes or until meat is no longer pink and thermometer reads 165°F. Remove from oven.

4 Spread marinara sauce evenly over cooked meat. Sprinkle mozzarella over sauce and top with pepperoni slices. Return to oven and bake until cheese is melted and bubbly, about 5 minutes.

PER SERVING

Calories: 410
Fat: 24g
Protein: 32g
Sodium: 1,068mg
Fiber: 2g
Carbohydrates: 11g
Net Carbohydrates: 9g
Sugar: 5g

BUNLESS BACON BURGERS

SERVES 2

The combination of avocado and mayonnaise in this recipe is so good you won't even miss the bun. For a handheld burger, serve these in large lettuce leaves for easier holding. For an even more decadent treat, add a fried egg on top and make sure to top it with plenty of keto-approved ketchup and mustard. Tessemae's and Primal Kitchen make delicious, no-sugar-added options.

½ pound 80/20 ground beef

2 tablespoons heavy cream

⅛ teaspoon hot pepper sauce

1 clove garlic, minced

1 tablespoon chopped onion

⅛ teaspoon black pepper

⅛ teaspoon salt

2 slices American cheese

2 slices no-sugar-added bacon, cooked

½ medium avocado, peeled, pitted, and sliced

1 tablespoon keto-friendly mayonnaise

1 Turn oven on to broil.

2 Place beef in a large mixing bowl and add heavy cream, hot sauce, garlic, onion, pepper, and salt. Mix until combined.

3 Form into four patties and place on a broiling rack. Broil 4 minutes on each side or until beef is no longer pink.

4 Top each burger with 1 slice American cheese and leave under broiler for 1 more minute.

5 Remove from oven and top each burger with 1 slice bacon and a quarter of sliced avocado. Drizzle ½ table-spoon mayonnaise onto each burger. Serve.

PER SERVING
Calories: 458
Fat: 33g
Protein: 27g
Sodium: 721mg
Fiber: 2g
Carbohydrates: 7g
Net Carbohydrates: 5g
Sugar: 2g

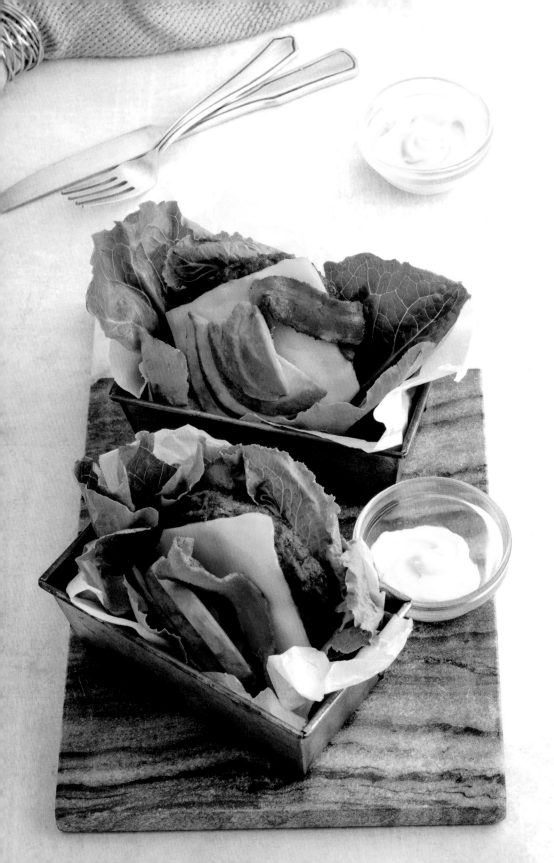

GORGONZOLA STEAK SALAD

SERVES 2

The combination of Gorgonzola crumbles and blue cheese dressing makes this salad taste like a decadent treat. Check your dressing labels diligently, and make sure you find a blue cheese that doesn't contain any added sugar or it will negatively affect the carb count.

1 tablespoon olive oil

½ pound sirloin steak

½ teaspoon salt

¼ teaspoon black pepper

4 cups mixed greens

2 large hard-boiled eggs, chopped

½ cup crumbled Gorgonzola cheese

¼ cup blue cheese dressing

1 In a large skillet over medium-high heat, heat olive oil. While oil is heating, rub steak with salt and pepper. Place steak in hot skillet and cook until desired doneness, about 4 minutes on each side for medium-rare, 7 minutes on each side for medium, and 9 minutes on each side for well-done. Set aside and let rest 10 minutes.

2 Put mixed greens in a large mixing bowl and top with hard-boiled eggs and crumbled Gorgonzola cheese.

3 Slice steak into thin strips and put on top of greens. Add dressing and toss until coated. Serve immediately.

PER SERVING

Calories: 589
Fat: 46g
Protein: 32g
Sodium: 1,286mg
Fiber: 1g
Carbohydrates: 5g
Net Carbohydrates: 4g
Sugar: 1g

THE CARBS IN GORGONZOLA

The flavor of Gorgonzola cheese is so strong that a little goes a long way. That's true for the fat content too. One half cup of the cheese contains 16 grams of fat, but only 0.5 net carbohydrates, making Gorgonzola cheese a good way to add some fat to any salad or even to a steak dish.

CHEESEBURGER SALAD

SERVES 2

This Cheeseburger Salad gives you all the characteristic flavors of a cheeseburger without the insulin- and glucose-spiking bun. It's perfect for a dinner partner who's missing a good burger but doesn't want to get kicked out of ketosis. If you don't have pickle juice, you can use white or apple cider vinegar in its place.

½ pound 85/15 ground beef

¼ teaspoon salt

⅛ teaspoon black pepper

3 tablespoons no-sugar-added ketchup

1 teaspoon yellow mustard

½ teaspoon spicy brown mustard

4 cups chopped romaine lettuce

2 tablespoons minced red onion

1 medium tomato, diced

2 dill pickle spears, cubed

½ cup shredded Cheddar cheese

4 tablespoons keto-friendly mayonnaise

2 teaspoons pickle juice

PER SERVING

Calories: 613
Fat: 46g
Protein: 38g
Sodium: 877mg
Fiber: 2g
Carbohydrates: 8g
Net Carbohydrates: 6g
Sugar: 4g

1 In a medium skillet over medium heat, brown ground beef. Once beef is browned, add salt, pepper, ketchup, yellow mustard, and spicy mustard. Stir until combined. Remove from heat and set aside.

2 Chop romaine lettuce and put into a large mixing bowl. Top with onions, tomatoes, pickles, cheese, and beef.

3 In a separate small bowl, combine mayonnaise with pickle juice and stir until smooth. Drizzle over salad and toss to coat. Serve immediately.

HYDRATE WITH PICKLE JUICE

When you think of hydration, your brain probably immediately goes to water, but pickle juice may actually be a better choice. Unlike plain water, which doesn't contain any electrolytes, pickle juice offers sodium and potassium. If you choose the right kind, the juice (or brine) also contains beneficial probiotics that can keep your gut healthy. Choose pickles that are refrigerated, naturally fermented, and don't contain any added dyes or artificial ingredients.

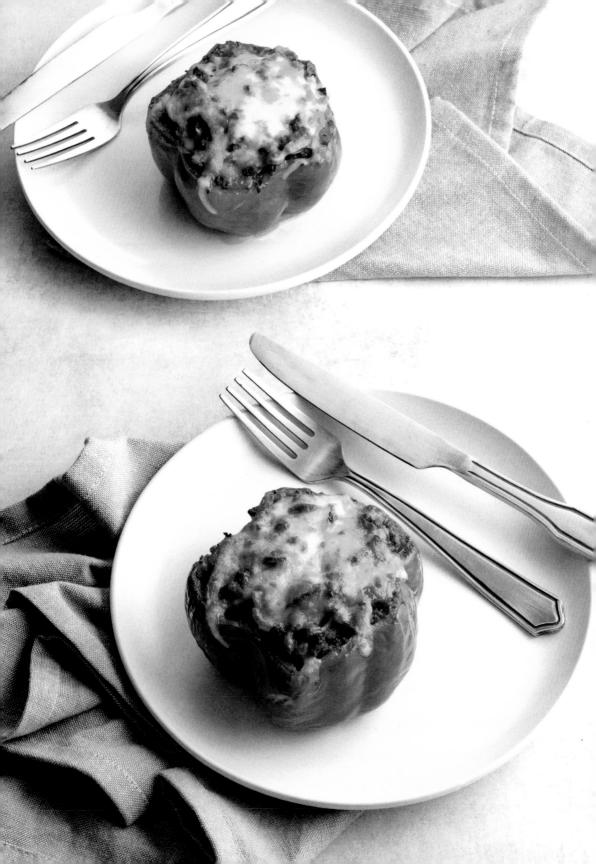

STUFFED GREEN PEPPERS

SERVES 2

You can swap the green peppers in this recipe for red peppers or yellow peppers if you prefer the taste, but keep in mind that this will change the carbohydrate count a little bit.

2 medium green bell peppers

1 tablespoon extra-virgin olive oil

¼ cup chopped yellow onion

1 clove garlic, minced

½ pound 85/15 ground beef

2 slices no-sugar-added bacon, cooked and diced

1 small tomato, diced

1 teaspoon Italian seasoning

2 tablespoons no-sugar-added marinara sauce

¼ cup shredded mozzarella cheese

¼ cup shredded Cheddar cheese

1 Preheat oven to 375°F.

2 Cut tops off bell peppers and remove seeds. Set aside.

3 In a large skillet over medium heat, heat olive oil and then sauté onion and garlic until transparent, about 5 minutes.

4 Add beef to skillet and cook until browned. Add bacon, tomato, and Italian seasoning and combine. Stir in marinara sauce.

5 Stuff each pepper with half of meat mixture and stand peppers upright in a baking pan. Bake 50 minutes or until meat reaches an internal temperature of 165°F.

6 Turn oven to broil and sprinkle cheeses on top of meat mixture. Broil 5 minutes or until cheese is melted and bubbly and peppers start to char. Remove from oven and serve hot.

PER SERVING
Calories: 529
Fat: 32g
Protein: 43g
Sodium: 480mg
Fiber: 4g
Carbohydrates: 14g
Net Carbohydrates: 10g
Sugar: 7g

THE CARBOHYDRATES IN PEPPERS

Bell peppers come in a variety of colors from green to yellow to red to orange, but you may not know that they all come from the same plant. A green bell pepper is the most immature version or, in other words, the least ripe. A red bell pepper is one that's been allowed to fully ripen. Yellow and orange bell peppers fall somewhere in between. Because the sugar content changes as the peppers get more ripe, red bell peppers are slightly higher in carbs than green ones, containing 5 grams and 4 grams of net carbs, respectively.

CHAPTER 9

SEAFOOD AND FISH MAIN DISHES

Omega-3 fatty acids are incredibly important for your heart and brain, yet a lot of Americans don't get enough in their diet. This is a big problem because your body lacks the ability to make omega-3s on its own, and the foods you eat are its only source. Enter seafood. Fatty fish, like salmon, are one of the richest sources of omega-3s (followed by plants, like flaxseed).

This chapter helps you optimize your fat intake by providing you with recipes that can easily and deliciously boost the amount of omega-3s you're eating. You'll use salmon in recipes like Smoked Salmon and Crème Fraîche Rollups and Baked Salmon with Garlic Aioli. You'll also find recipes for crab, shrimp, and tuna.

When choosing a tuna, it's a good idea to opt for brands that responsibly source theirs by fishing with poles instead of nets. One brand, called Safe Catch, also tests its tuna for mercury, so you'll know the tuna you're eating isn't just keto-approved; it's safe too.

SMOKED SALMON AND CRÈME FRAÎCHE ROLLUPS

SERVES 2

If you love a bagel and lox for breakfast or Sunday brunch, try these Smoked Salmon and Crème Fraîche Rollups instead. They will be just as satisfying, but even more rewarding, since you'll get all the flavor without any of the carbs. If you want an even more authentic bagel taste, sprinkle some everything bagel seasoning on top.

4 ounces crème fraîche

¼ teaspoon fresh lemon zest

4 (1-ounce) slices smoked salmon

1 In a small bowl, mix crème fraîche and lemon zest.

2 Spread a quarter of mixture on top of each salmon slice.

3 Roll slices into individual rolls and secure with a toothpick. Serve immediately.

PER SERVING
Calories: 273
Fat: 23g
Protein: 12g
Sodium: 1,152mg
Fiber: 0g
Carbohydrates: 2g
Net Carbohydrates: 2g
Sugar: 2g

CRAB AND AVOCADO ENDIVE CUPS

SERVES 2

The crab in these Crab and Avocado Endive Cups gives a slightly sweet taste to the dish without adding a single carbohydrate. If you want to add a little more fat, you can drizzle any of the keto-approved Tessemae's dressings on top of the filling after stuffing the endive.

1 (6-ounce) can crabmeat, drained

1 large avocado, peeled, pitted, and chopped

2 tablespoons finely chopped cilantro

⅓ cup chopped green onion

2 tablespoons fresh lime juice

⅓ cup coconut oil

½ teaspoon sea salt

¼ teaspoon freshly ground black pepper

8 Belgian endive leaves

1 In a small food processor, mix all ingredients except endive until well blended.

2 Evenly divide crab mix onto each endive cup. Serve immediately.

PER SERVING
Calories: 489
Fat: 44g
Protein: 13g
Sodium: 740mg
Fiber: 6g
Carbohydrates: 9g
Net Carbohydrates: 3g
Sugar: 1g

CREAMY TUNA ENDIVE CUPS

SERVES 2

Like crab, tuna contains virtually no carbohydrates. Because of that, it's an excellent choice for this endive cup variation. These Creamy Tuna Endive Cups are a super-simple, super-quick recipe that you can make for two in just a few minutes.

1 (5-ounce) can tuna in olive oil, drained

5 ounces cream cheese

8 Belgian endive leaves

4 tablespoons hemp hearts

1 In a small food processor, mix tuna and cream cheese until well blended.

2 Evenly divide the tuna cream onto each endive cup.

3 Sprinkle ½ tablespoon hemp hearts over each endive cup. Serve immediately.

PER SERVING
Calories: 411
Fat: 32g
Protein: 19g
Sodium: 376mg
Fiber: 1g
Carbohydrates: 5g
Net Carbohydrates: 4g
Sugar: 2g

HEMP HEARTS

Hemp hearts is the term used for shelled hemp seeds. These little seeds contain 30 percent fat, most of which is in the form of alpha-linolenic acid, an omega-3 fatty acid, and linoleic acid, an omega-6 fatty acid. These fats have been shown to reduce the risk of heart disease and keep your skin healthy. Hemp hearts are also rich in both protein and fiber, so you can up the nutritional content of any meal by sprinkling a little bit of hemp on top.

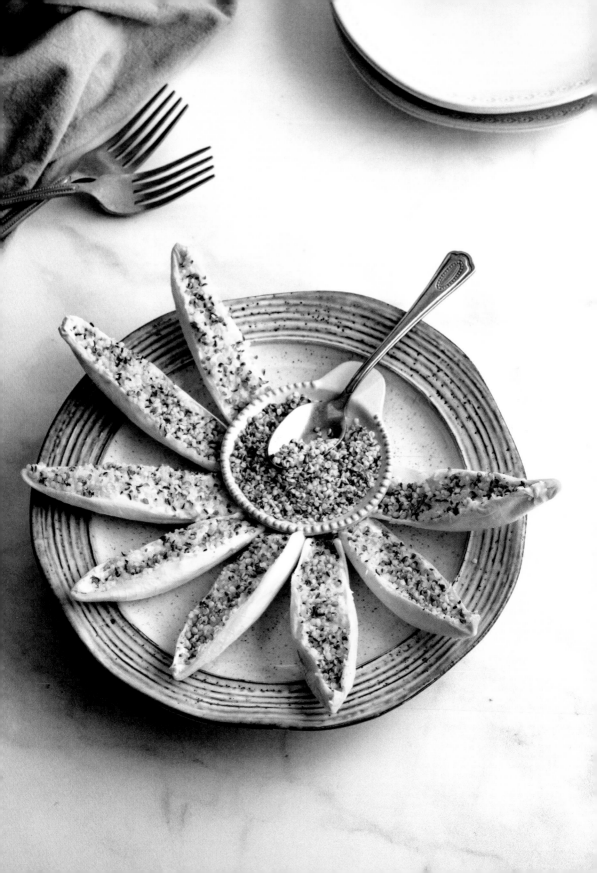

TUNA AND EGG SALAD

SERVES 2

This recipe is designed for two, but if you want to save time later, you can double or triple it and store the Tuna and Egg Salad in the refrigerator for your lunches the next day. Serve with sliced raw zucchini or cucumber slices.

2 large hard-boiled eggs

1 (5-ounce) can tuna packed in water

¼ cup olive oil mayonnaise

¼ cup diced white onion

¼ cup no-sugar-added relish

¼ teaspoon salt

¼ teaspoon black pepper

1 Put eggs in a medium mixing bowl and mash with a fork.

2 Add tuna and mayonnaise and mash together until ingredients are combined. Stir in onion, relish, salt, and pepper. Serve.

PER SERVING

Calories: 297	Fiber: 1g
Fat: 16g	Carbohydrates: 15g
Protein: 20g	Net Carbohydrates: 14g
Sodium: 1,110mg	Sugar: 1g

STUFFED AVOCADOS

SERVES 2

Avocados top the list of keto dieters' favorites because they're rich in monounsaturated fats and fiber, so the net carbohydrates are low. When making this recipe, it's best to choose avocados that are ripe but still firm. If the avocados are too soft, they'll be too mushy and won't hold the tuna as well.

1 large avocado

1 (5-ounce) can tuna packed in water

2 tablespoons keto-friendly mayonnaise

½ medium green bell pepper, seeded and chopped

¼ teaspoon dried minced onion

⅛ teaspoon garlic salt

⅛ teaspoon black pepper

1 Cut avocado in half lengthwise and remove the pit. Set aside.

2 In a medium mixing bowl, put tuna, mayonnaise, bell pepper, dried onion, garlic salt, and pepper and mash together with a fork until combined.

3 Scoop half of the mixture into each half of the avocado. Serve.

PER SERVING

Calories: 292	Fiber: 5g
Fat: 23g	Carbohydrates: 7g
Protein: 15g	Net Carbohydrates: 2g
Sodium: 416mg	Sugar: 1g

CRAB DYNAMITE-BAKED AVOCADOS

SERVES 2

Looking for an easy way to prepare sushi for two? This recipe has got you covered. It's an at-home version of the dish Dynamite that's popular in some American sushi restaurants. It uses avocado, keto-approved mayonnaise, and crabmeat, three excellent choices for a keto diet.

2 medium avocados, halved and pitted, skin on

3 ounces real crabmeat, drained from juices

4 teaspoons keto-friendly mayonnaise

2 teaspoons coconut aminos or tamari

½ teaspoon freshly ground black pepper

1 Preheat oven to 350°F.

2 Place avocado halves hole side up in a shallow ramekin or ovenproof dish just large enough to hold them.

3 In a small bowl, mix crabmeat, mayonnaise, coconut aminos, and pepper, then divide and scoop into each avocado cavity.

4 Bake 20 minutes. Serve hot.

PER SERVING

Calories: 336
Fat: 27g
Protein: 10g
Sodium: 298mg
Fiber: 9g
Carbohydrates: 13g
Net Carbohydrates: 4g
Sugar: 0g

SOY-FREE COCONUT AMINOS

Coconut aminos is a great substitution for soy sauce for people who prefer not using any soy products. It has a similar taste, but comes from coconut sap and is completely soy- and additive-free. As the popularity of keto grows, ingredients like coconut aminos have become more readily available. You can purchase it from many major retailers online and in stores now.

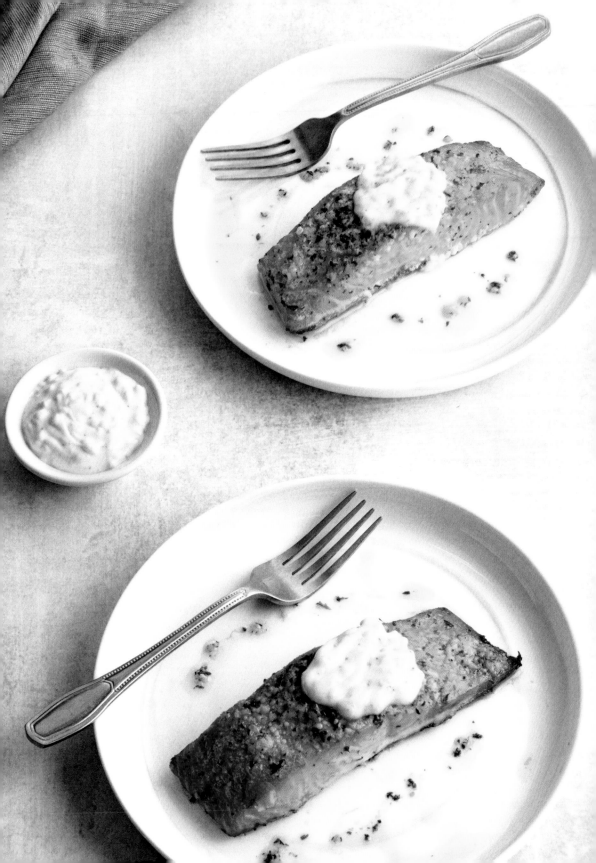

BAKED SALMON WITH GARLIC AIOLI

SERVES 2

Watch the clock when marinating this recipe. If you leave raw fish sitting in lemon juice too long, the fish will start to "cook." The citric acid in the lemon juice can change the proteins in the fish, turning the flesh firm and opaque, similar to how it would look and feel if it had been cooked with heat.

FOR GARLIC AIOLI

½ cup olive oil mayonnaise

2 cloves garlic, minced

1½ tablespoons olive oil

1 tablespoon fresh lemon juice

¼ teaspoon salt

⅛ teaspoon black pepper

FOR SALMON

1½ cloves garlic, minced

2 tablespoons extra-virgin olive oil

2 tablespoons melted grass-fed butter

½ tablespoon lemon juice

¼ teaspoon salt

¼ teaspoon black pepper

½ teaspoon dried parsley

2 (6-ounce) salmon fillets

1 To make garlic aioli: Mix all ingredients together in a small bowl until smooth. Cover and refrigerate.

2 To make salmon: Combine garlic, olive oil, butter, lemon juice, salt, pepper, and parsley in a medium mixing bowl. Place salmon in a baking pan and pour marinade on top. Refrigerate 1 hour.

3 Preheat oven to 350°F.

4 Put salmon in oven and bake 35 minutes or until fish flakes easily with a fork.

5 Remove from oven and top each piece of salmon with garlic aioli, evenly dividing the aioli between each piece.

OUTSTANDING OMEGA-3S

A 4-ounce fillet of salmon contains just about 15 grams of fat. Most of this fat comes in the form of omega-3 fatty acids, which promote brain health and heart health and help protect against cancer and autoimmune diseases such as rheumatoid arthritis and lupus. When you're looking to up your fat intake for the day in a healthy way, salmon is a great choice.

PER SERVING

Calories: 742
Fat: 60g
Protein: 35g
Sodium: 1,164mg
Fiber: 0g
Carbohydrates: 7g
Net Carbohydrates: 7g
Sugar: 0g

SALMON AND AVOCADO SALAD

SERVES 2

Instead of serving this salmon and avocado combo as a salad, you can spread the cream cheese mixture on each piece of smoked salmon and roll it up instead. Either way, it makes a perfectly balanced keto meal for two.

2 ounces cream cheese, softened

2 tablespoons extra-virgin olive oil

⅛ teaspoon salt

2 teaspoons lemon juice

8 ounces smoked salmon, chopped

2 large avocados, peeled, pitted, and cubed

1 In a food processor or blender, put cream cheese, olive oil, salt, and lemon juice and process until smooth.

2 In a medium bowl, add smoked salmon to avocado and toss in cream cheese dressing. Refrigerate until chilled, 30 minutes to 1 hour. Serve chilled.

PER SERVING
Calories: 578
Fat: 45g
Protein: 25g
Sodium: 2,528mg
Fiber: 9g
Carbohydrates: 13g
Net Carbohydrates: 4g
Sugar: 1g

KALE AND SALMON SALAD

SERVES 2

Baby kale is not as tough as regular kale, and it has a milder taste too. If you're not a big kale lover, try baby kale before knocking it completely. If you want to soften it even more, massage the kale with a little extra lemon juice before adding the rest of the ingredients on top.

6 tablespoons olive oil, divided

2 cloves garlic, minced

1 (8-ounce) salmon fillet

½ teaspoon salt

¼ teaspoon black pepper

1 tablespoon lemon juice

4 cups chopped baby kale

1 large avocado, peeled, pitted, and diced

2 tablespoons pine nuts

2 tablespoons apple cider vinegar

PER SERVING
Calories: 696
Fat: 57g
Protein: 27g
Sodium: 684mg
Fiber: 6g
Carbohydrates: 12g
Net Carbohydrates: 6g
Sugar: 2g

1 In a large skillet over medium heat, heat 2 tablespoons olive oil. Add garlic and sauté 3 minutes.

2 Season salmon with salt and pepper and add to hot pan. Cook 4 minutes on each side or until fish flakes easily with a fork. Drizzle lemon juice on top. Remove from heat.

3 Divide kale between two plates and top each plate with half of avocado, 1 tablespoon pine nuts, and 4 ounces salmon.

4 In a separate small bowl, combine remaining 4 tablespoons olive oil and apple cider vinegar. Pour half of mixture over each plate.

HAIL THE KALE

Kale has earned its top spot as a nutrition superfood, and for good reason. The low-carb veggie is one of the best dietary sources of vitamin K, which keeps your blood healthy, and is loaded with antioxidants that help reduce your risk of chronic diseases, like cancer. Kale is also rich in vitamin A, vitamin C, manganese, and beta-carotene. If you don't like regular kale, try to at least include some baby kale in your diet to reap all the benefits of the cruciferous vegetable.

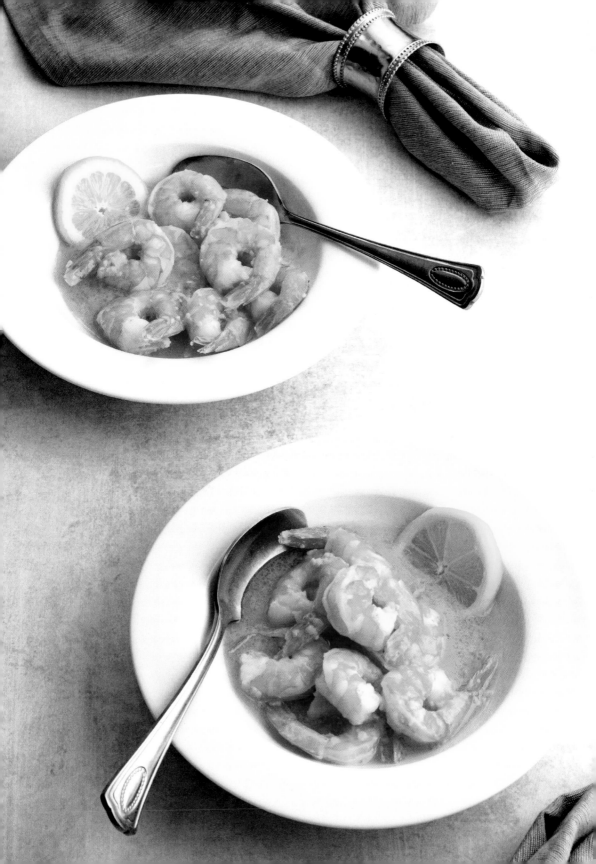

SHRIMP SCAMPI

SERVES 2

Don't be intimated by shrimp. This dish is easy to prepare and extremely versatile. Pour it over zucchini noodles or a plate of spinach. If you have room for a few extra carbohydrates, try spooning it over roasted spaghetti squash instead.

½ pound cooked medium shrimp

6 tablespoons grass-fed butter

1 clove garlic, minced

2 teaspoons lemon juice

PER SERVING
Calories: 467
Fat: 38g
Protein: 26g
Sodium: 1,178mg
Fiber: 0g
Carbohydrates: 3g
Net Carbohydrates: 3g
Sugar: 0g

1 Remove tails from shrimp. Set shrimp aside.

2 In a large skillet over medium heat, melt butter. When butter is hot, add garlic and sauté until translucent, 3–4 minutes.

3 Add lemon juice and shrimp and cook until shrimp is hot, about 2 minutes. Serve shrimp with garlic butter poured on top.

BENEFITS OF SHRIMP

Shrimp is an unusually concentrated source of the carotenoid astaxanthin, which acts as an antioxidant and an anti-inflammatory agent that helps fight free radicals and protect you from chronic diseases, like cancer and heart disease. It's also an excellent source of the mineral selenium, which keeps your thyroid healthy and is lacking in many Americans' diets.

CHAPTER 10

VEGETARIAN MAIN DISHES

Don't ever let anyone tell you that you can't do keto if you're vegetarian! With these low-carb, keto-approved recipes, you can stay within your macronutrient ranges without eating any meat, and you'll enjoy it too. This chapter provides recipes with plenty of plant-based fats, like avocado and olives, as well as all types of cheeses, like cream cheese, ricotta, and feta cheese. But if you, or the person you're sharing your meal with, are vegan, you can easily skip the cheese.

Even if your dining partner isn't vegetarian, or you're just trying to incorporate more Meatless Mondays, you'll both enjoy everything this chapter has to offer. Try the Stuffed Portobello Mushrooms or go for the Zoodles with Avocado Pesto instead. Whip up some Ricotta-Stuffed Eggplant or put together some Mediterranean Rollups, perfectly designed for two.

AVOCADO AND WALNUT SALAD

SERVES 2

If you want to up the fat content of this Avocado and Walnut Salad a bit, you can sprinkle some feta, blue cheese, or Gorgonzola cheese crumbles on top. Serve it with a drizzle of Tessemae's Avocado Ranch or use Green Goddess dressing if you want something less creamy.

---

1 small lime

2 large avocados, peeled, pitted, and cubed

⅔ cup walnut pieces

⅓ cup cherry tomatoes, halved

⅛ cup sliced black olives

1 tablespoon extra-virgin olive oil

⅛ teaspoon salt

⅛ teaspoon black pepper

In a large bowl, squeeze juice from lime over avocados. Add remaining ingredients and toss until combined. Serve.

PER SERVING

Calories: 568
Fat: 52g
Protein: 9g
Sodium: 222mg

Fiber: 12g
Carbohydrates: 19g
Net Carbohydrates: 7g
Sugar: 2g

STUFFED PORTOBELLO MUSHROOMS

SERVES 2

You can easily change the flavor of this recipe by using blue cheese, Gorgonzola cheese, or goat cheese in place of feta. If you prefer to make it vegan, lose the cheese completely and use some nutritional yeast—which only contains 1 gram of net carbohydrates per 2 tablespoon serving—instead.

---

4 large portobello mushrooms

½ cup crumbled feta cheese

1 cup chopped fresh spinach

2 tablespoons chopped fresh oregano

1 tablespoon extra-virgin olive oil

1 Preheat oven to 350°F.

2 Remove stems from mushrooms and chop stems into small pieces. Put chopped stems, feta, spinach, and oregano in a medium bowl and toss to combine.

3 Brush each mushroom inside and out with olive oil and then stuff with feta mixture. Put on a baking rack and bake 20 minutes or until mushroom is soft and cheese is melted.

PER SERVING

Calories: 198
Fat: 14g
Protein: 9g
Sodium: 370mg

Fiber: 3g
Carbohydrates: 9g
Net Carbohydrates: 6g
Sugar: 6g

CREAMY SPAGHETTI SQUASH

SERVES 2

If you want to reduce the carbohydrate count of this dish a little more, replace the spaghetti squash with lightly sautéed (or even raw) zucchini noodles. A cup of spaghetti squash contains 5.5 grams of net carbs, while the same serving size of zucchini contains only 2.7 grams.

½ small spaghetti squash

3 tablespoons olive oil, divided

¼ teaspoon salt

⅓ cup cream cheese

2 tablespoons sour cream

¼ cup full-fat canned coconut milk

¼ cup heavy cream

2 tablespoons grated vegetarian Parmesan cheese

1 tablespoon grated Asiago cheese

¼ teaspoon onion powder

½ teaspoon dried chives

1 Preheat oven to 400°F.

2 Carefully cut spaghetti squash in half lengthwise and scoop out the seeds. Brush 2 tablespoons olive oil over flesh of squash and sprinkle salt on top. Place on baking sheet, cut side up, and bake 45 minutes or until squash is fork tender.

3 Scrape squash out of shell with a fork and put in a medium bowl.

4 In a medium saucepan over medium heat, add remaining 1 tablespoon olive oil. Add cream cheese and stir until melted. Add sour cream, coconut milk, heavy cream, cheeses, and onion powder to saucepan, stirring frequently until sauce is bubbling.

5 Remove from heat and pour over spaghetti squash. Toss to coat. Sprinkle chives on top. Serve.

PER SERVING

Calories: 565
Fat: 51g
Protein: 7g
Sodium: 599mg
Fiber: 2g
Carbohydrates: 15g
Net Carbohydrates: 13g
Sugar: 6g

KEEP AN EYE OUT

Be careful not to overcook spaghetti squash. When you do, the flesh turns mushy, loses its spaghetti-like quality, and resembles a mashed vegetable dish instead of noodles. Cook it just until tender, let it cool slightly, and then remove strands from the skin with a fork.

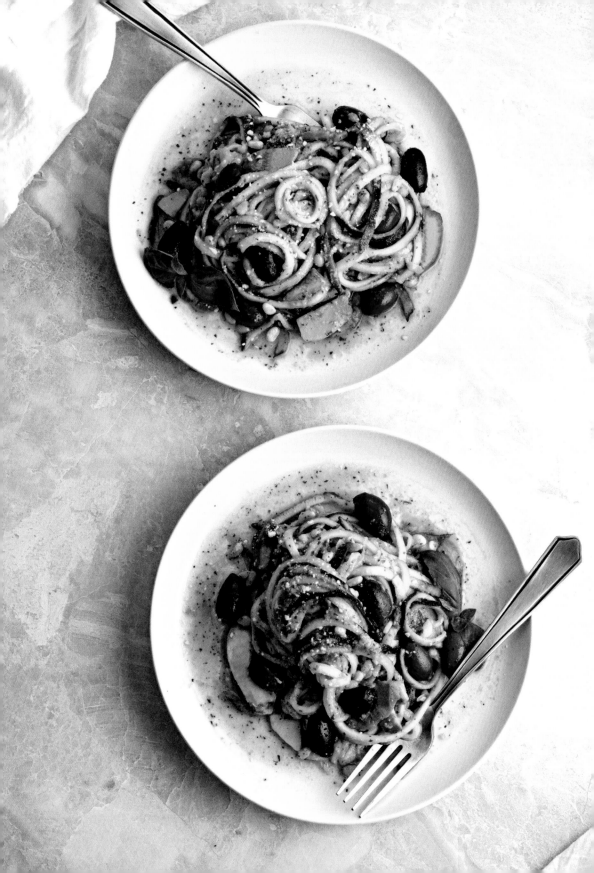

ZOODLES WITH AVOCADO PESTO

SERVES 2

Traditionally, pesto is made with pine nuts, but for a different, nuttier flavor you can replace the pine nuts in this recipe with raw, unsalted walnuts. That will actually reduce the carbohydrate count a little too. One-fourth cup of pine nuts has 3.25 grams of net carbohydrates, while the same serving of walnuts has 2 grams of net carbs.

2 large zucchini

2 medium avocados, divided

1 cup chopped fresh basil

2 teaspoons lemon juice

1 clove garlic

¼ cup plus 1 tablespoon extra-virgin olive oil, divided

¼ teaspoon salt

¼ teaspoon black pepper

¼ cup grated vegetarian Parmesan cheese

¼ cup pine nuts

½ cup kalamata olives

1 Cut zucchini into long strips using a vegetable peeler or a spiralizer. Set zucchini "noodles" aside on a paper towel and allow them to sweat.

2 Peel one avocado, remove the pit, and scoop out flesh. Add avocado to a blender, along with basil, lemon juice, garlic, ¼ cup olive oil, salt, pepper, and Parmesan cheese and process until smooth.

3 In a large skillet over medium heat, heat remaining 1 tablespoon olive oil. Add zucchini noodles and sauté until softened, but still firm, about 4 minutes.

4 Pour sauce into skillet, along with pine nuts and olives, and toss to coat zucchini.

5 Remove from heat. Slice remaining avocado and add to zucchini mixture. Toss to combine. Serve.

PER SERVING

Calories: 856
Fat: 77g
Protein: 13g
Sodium: 1,242mg
Fiber: 13g
Carbohydrates: 27g
Net Carbohydrates: 14g
Sugar: 9g

SHOW OLIVES SOME LOVE

The monounsaturated fats found in olives have been shown to encourage weight loss by breaking down the fats inside your fat cells and reducing insulin sensitivity. At only 1 gram of carbohydrates for five olives, they are a perfect ketogenic diet snack, salad topping, or taco bowl addition.

CAULIFLOWER CASSEROLE

SERVES 2

If you prefer a thicker casserole, you can replace half of the sour cream in this recipe with equal parts softened cream cheese. The cream cheese doesn't change the carb count much, but it does hold the Cauliflower Casserole together a little more.

3 cups cauliflower florets

2 tablespoons heavy cream

1 tablespoon grass-fed butter

⅛ teaspoon garlic powder

⅛ teaspoon onion powder

⅛ teaspoon paprika

¼ teaspoon salt

¼ teaspoon black pepper

¾ cup shredded Cheddar cheese, divided

¼ cup fire-roasted diced tomatoes

¼ cup sour cream

1 tablespoon diced fresh jalapeños

¼ cup sliced black olives

PER SERVING
Calories: 413
Fat: 32g
Protein: 15g
Sodium: 837mg
Fiber: 4g
Carbohydrates: 12g
Net Carbohydrates: 8g
Sugar: 5g

1 Preheat oven to 350°F.

2 Bring a large pot of water to a boil and add cauliflower florets. Boil until fork tender, about 8 minutes.

3 Drain and transfer cauliflower to a food processor or blender. Add heavy cream, butter, garlic powder, onion powder, paprika, salt, and pepper and process until smooth. Add ¼ cup cheese and stir until combined.

4 Pour cauliflower mixture into a 9" × 5" baking pan and spread out evenly. Spread diced tomatoes on top of cauliflower and sour cream on top of tomatoes. Sprinkle with remaining cheese, jalapeños, and olives.

5 Bake 45 minutes or until cheese is melted and casserole is bubbling. Allow to cool before serving.

HALF-AND-HALF OR HEAVY CREAM?

Many people on a keto diet shun half-and-half, which is made up of half heavy cream and half whole milk, because the milk adds a touch of natural sugar. But the fears surrounding half-and-half are unnecessary. While 2 tablespoons of half-and-half contain 1.2 grams of carbohydrates, heavy cream offers 0.8 grams. Not too far off. If you prefer to use half-and-half over heavy cream, that's usually okay. Just make sure you're aware that it does slightly change the carbohydrate count.

VEGETABLE OMELET

SERVES 2

Eggs and vegetables are the perfect pair on a keto diet. The eggs provide healthy fats, protein, and various vitamins and minerals, and nonstarchy veggies provide fiber without adding a lot of carbs. Make this Vegetable Omelet as written, or throw in your favorite combo of veggies to make it your own.

1 tablespoon coconut oil

2 tablespoons chopped white onion

½ cup diced zucchini

2 tablespoons diced green bell pepper

1 cup fresh spinach

4 large eggs

2 tablespoons heavy cream

⅛ teaspoon salt

⅛ teaspoon black pepper

¼ cup shredded Cheddar cheese

1 small avocado, peeled, pitted, and chopped

PER SERVING

Calories: 437
Fat: 34g
Protein: 19g
Sodium: 401mg
Fiber: 6g
Carbohydrates: 10g
Net Carbohydrates: 4g
Sugar: 3g

1 In a large skillet over medium heat, heat coconut oil. When skillet is hot, add onions, zucchini, and bell pepper. Sauté until soft, about 5 minutes. Add spinach and sauté until wilted.

2 In a medium bowl, whisk eggs, heavy cream, salt, and black pepper together.

3 Pour egg mixture over sautéed vegetables and cook 2–3 minutes or until eggs begin to set. Lift the edges of the eggs with a spatula and tilt the skillet so that uncooked egg moves to the side of the pan. Continue cooking about 3 minutes or until egg is almost fully set.

4 Add cheese to half of the egg and flip the other side over with a spatula.

5 Let the omelet cook 2–3 more minutes or until cheese is melted. Remove from heat and top with chopped avocado.

BAKED ZUCCHINI

SERVES 2

This Baked Zucchini dish gives traditional lasagna a run for its money. You can increase the amount of vitamins, minerals, and antioxidants in it by adding some mushrooms and sautéed spinach or whatever low-carb vegetables the two of you enjoy.

1 tablespoon extra-virgin olive oil

¼ cup chopped yellow onion

2 medium zucchini, julienned

¾ cup shredded mozzarella cheese, divided

¼ cup full-fat ricotta cheese

1 tablespoon cream cheese

¾ cup sugar-free marinara sauce

1 clove garlic, minced

2 tablespoons chopped fresh basil

2 tablespoons chopped fresh oregano

¼ teaspoon salt

¼ teaspoon black pepper

1 Preheat oven to 350°F.

2 In a large skillet over medium heat, heat olive oil and add onion. Sauté until translucent, about 3 minutes, then add zucchini. Sauté another 4 minutes or until zucchini is softened but still firm.

3 Add ½ cup mozzarella cheese, ricotta cheese, cream cheese, marinara, garlic, basil, oregano, salt, and pepper to the pan. Bring to a simmer and remove from heat once cream cheese is melted.

4 Transfer to a 5" × 9" baking pan. Top with remaining mozzarella and bake 15 minutes or until cheese is melted and casserole is bubbling.

PER SERVING
Calories: 339
Fat: 22g
Protein: 19g
Sodium: 823mg
Fiber: 4g
Carbohydrates: 19g
Net Carbohydrates: 15g
Sugar: 11g

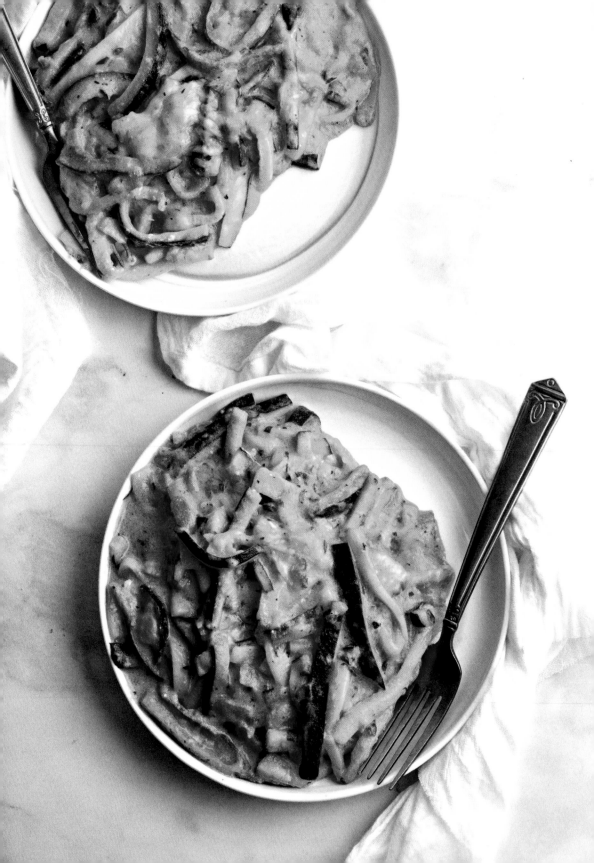

MEDITERRANEAN ROLLUPS

SERVES 2

Extra-virgin olive oil and kalamata olives come together in this recipe to give you heaps of oleic acid, a type of monounsaturated fat that can help reduce inflammation and may even reduce your risk of developing certain types of cancer. Finish these rollups off with a few crumbles of feta cheese if you want.

2 large eggs, divided

2 tablespoons extra-virgin olive oil, divided

¼ teaspoon sea salt, divided

12 large kalamata olives, pitted

2 ounces sun-dried tomatoes in oil

¼ teaspoon red chili flakes

¼ teaspoon parsley flakes

PER SERVING
Calories: 303
Fat: 27g
Protein: 8g
Sodium: 686mg
Fiber: 2g
Carbohydrates: 7g
Net Carbohydrates: 5g
Sugar: 0g

1 In a small bowl, combine one egg, 1 tablespoon olive oil, and ⅛ teaspoon salt and whisk until foamy.

2 Heat a small nonstick skillet over high heat and pour in egg mixture, spreading evenly so it forms a thin, even layer.

3 Once the first side is cooked, about 1 minute, flip with the aid of a plate or a lid. Cook until golden on bottom, about 2 more minutes.

4 Remove frittata to a plate.

5 Repeat the above steps with remaining egg, olive oil, and salt.

6 In a food processor, mix olives, tomatoes, chili flakes, and parsley flakes until well chopped and blended, about 30 seconds.

7 Equally divide olive paste between the frittatas, spreading it on top of each in an even layer.

8 Roll each frittata into a tight roll, and cut both in half. Serve immediately.

QUATTRO FORMAGGI ROLLUPS

SERVES 2

"Quattro Formaggi" is a fancy Italian term that translates simply to "four cheese." These Quattro Formaggi Rollups combine Parmesan, blue cheese, mascarpone, and Brie to give you a rich, fatty finished dish. If you or your dining partner prefers milder cheeses, you can swap any of these out for mozzarella, provolone, or even Cheddar.

2 large eggs, divided

2 tablespoons grated vegetarian Parmesan cheese, divided

2 tablespoons crumbled blue cheese, divided

2 tablespoons grass-fed butter, divided

2 tablespoons mascarpone cheese, divided

2 ounces thinly sliced Brie cheese, divided

PER SERVING
Calories: 379
Fat: 32g
Protein: 17g
Sodium: 458mg
Fiber: 0g
Carbohydrates: 3g
Net Carbohydrates: 3g
Sugar: 1g

1 In a small bowl, whisk one egg, 1 tablespoon Parmesan, and 1 tablespoon blue cheese until foamy.

2 Heat a small nonstick skillet over high heat and melt 1 tablespoon butter.

3 Pour in egg mixture, spreading evenly so it forms a thin, even layer.

4 Once the first side is cooked, about 1 minute, flip frittata with the aid of a plate or a lid.

5 Spread 1 tablespoon mascarpone on top of frittata, then place 1 ounce Brie slices in the middle and cover with a lid.

6 Cook until golden on bottom, about 2 more minutes.

7 Remove frittata to a plate.

8 Repeat steps with remaining ingredients.

9 Roll each frittata into a tight roll, cut into two pieces, and serve immediately while hot.

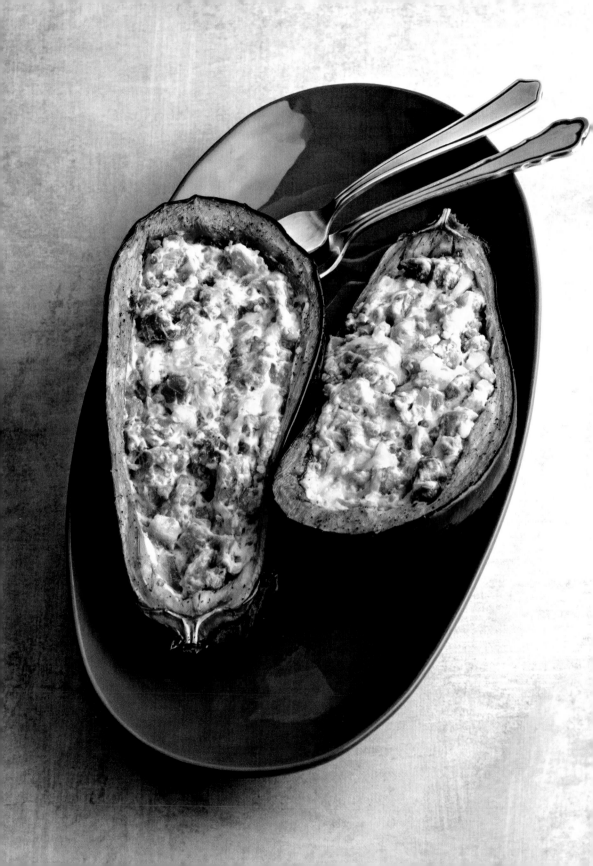

RICOTTA-STUFFED EGGPLANT

SERVES 2

The best eggplants are those that are firm and shiny without any broken skin. Smaller eggplants also tend to be less bitter than larger ones, so keep that in mind when choosing eggplants for this recipe. If you want the eggplant to be a little sweeter, pick small ones.

1 small eggplant

2 tablespoons extra-virgin olive oil, divided

¼ teaspoon salt

⅛ teaspoon black pepper

1 clove garlic, minced

1 tablespoon minced shallots

½ cup full-fat ricotta cheese

¼ cup shredded mozzarella cheese

PER SERVING
Calories: 340
Fat: 24g
Protein: 13g
Sodium: 423mg
Fiber: 8g
Carbohydrates: 20g
Net Carbohydrates: 12g
Sugar: 10g

1 Preheat oven to 350°F.

2 Cut eggplant in half and scoop out some of the insides to create a bowl. Brush bowls with 1 tablespoon olive oil and sprinkle with salt and pepper. Dice insides and set aside.

3 Place eggplant halves on a baking sheet, cut side up, and bake 20 minutes or until eggplant is soft.

4 While eggplant is baking, heat remaining 1 tablespoon olive oil in a medium skillet over medium heat. Add diced eggplant, garlic, and shallots to pan and sauté until soft, about 8 minutes. Remove from heat and allow to cool slightly.

5 In a large bowl, combine cooked eggplant, ricotta, and mozzarella cheese. When eggplants are done cooking, fill them with cheese mixture, and return to the oven for 10 minutes or until cheese is melted and bubbly.

MALE VERSUS FEMALE EGGPLANTS

Did you know that there are male and female eggplants? The male eggplants have fewer seeds than the female eggplants, so they tend to be less bitter. You can determine the sex of an eggplant by looking at the indentation on the bottom. If the indentation is shallow and round, it's a male; if the indentation is deep and more rectangular, it's a female.

DESSERTS

Do you want the good news or the bad news first? The bad news is that sugar is out on keto, so you probably won't find many store-bought desserts that fit within your carbohydrate needs. The good news is that with so many keto-approved sweeteners, like erythritol, stevia, and monk fruit, you'll be able to make two-serving keto-friendly desserts at home. The even better news is that, like artificial sweeteners, these types of sweeteners don't raise your blood sugar or insulin levels, but *unlike* artificial sweeteners, which have been linked to weight gain and inflammation, they don't come with any negative health effects.

The next time you're whipping up dinner for two, opt for one of the desserts in this chapter too. You'll find everything from Chocolate Chia Pudding to Lemon Mug Cake with Lemon Icing to Pistachio Pudding, so you can satisfy any type of craving.

LEMON MUG CAKE WITH LEMON ICING

SERVES 2

Don't skip the zest in this recipe! It may seem like a small addition, but it really enhances the lemon flavor. If you don't have lemon juice or zest, you can use a teeny bit of lemon extract in its place.

FOR LEMON MUG CAKE

¾ cup almond flour

3 tablespoons granulated erythritol

½ teaspoon baking powder

⅛ teaspoon salt

Juice and zest of 1 medium lemon

1 large egg

2 tablespoons grass-fed butter, melted

FOR LEMON ICING

2 tablespoons powdered erythritol

½ teaspoon water

½ teaspoon lemon juice

PER SERVING

Calories: 390
Fat: 35g
Protein: 12g
Sodium: 337mg
Fiber: 5g
Carbohydrates: 38g
Net Carbohydrates: 19.5g
Sugar: 2g

1 In a medium bowl, mix almond flour, granulated erythritol, baking powder, and salt together. Add lemon juice, lemon zest, egg, and melted butter and whisk until combined.

2 In a small bowl, mix powdered erythritol, water, and lemon juice together.

3 Divide almond flour mixture evenly between two microwave-safe mugs. Microwave on high for 90 seconds each.

4 Combine icing ingredients and drizzle on top of each mug cake. Serve warm.

ZEST AWAY

When zesting a lemon, remove only the yellow outer skin. The white part just under the yellow skin, which is called the pith, has a bitter taste that can be unpleasant, especially in sweet dishes. A special kitchen tool called a microplane is available to help make zesting easier, but you can do it with a regular grater if you're careful.

CHOCOLATE MUG CAKE

SERVES 2

When you're making dessert for two, the last thing you want to do is bake a whole cake or pan of brownies, since not eating the whole thing in one sitting takes some serious self-control. These Chocolate Mug Cakes are a great way to get your chocolate fix in a single serving size.

2 tablespoons unsalted butter, melted

3 tablespoons almond flour

1 tablespoon coconut flour

1 large egg

2 tablespoons granulated erythritol

¼ teaspoon vanilla extract

⅛ teaspoon salt

¾ teaspoon baking powder

1½ tablespoons unsweetened cocoa powder

1 tablespoon stevia-sweetened chocolate chips

1 Put all ingredients in a small bowl and whisk until smooth.

2 Split the batter evenly between two microwave-safe mugs. Microwave each mug on high for 75 seconds or until batter has set. Serve.

PER SERVING
Calories: 247
Fat: 21g
Protein: 8g
Sodium: 185mg
Fiber: 6g
Carbohydrates: 24g
Net Carbohydrates: 15g
Sugar: 3g

CHOCOLATE CHIA PUDDING

SERVES 2

Chia pudding is so simple and versatile you can make it with just about any combination of ingredients. Try sunflower butter in place of coconut butter and ½ cup brewed coffee in place of ½ cup coconut cream for some variations that don't change the carbohydrate count much.

1 cup full-fat coconut cream

3 tablespoons unsweetened cocoa powder

2 tablespoons granulated erythritol

¼ cup coconut butter

3 tablespoons chia seeds

1 Put all ingredients except chia seeds in a blender and blend until smooth.

2 Transfer to a sealable container and add chia seeds. Shake to combine.

3 Refrigerate 8 hours or until chia seeds have absorbed enough liquid to turn mixture into a pudding-like consistency. Serve chilled.

PER SERVING
Calories: 688
Fat: 63g
Protein: 10g
Sodium: 18mg
Fiber: 15g
Carbohydrates: 37g
Net Carbohydrates: 19g
Sugar: 2g

SUPER CHIA SEEDS

A single ounce of chia seeds contains 9 grams of fat (5 of which are omega-3s) and 4 grams of protein. There are 12 grams of carbohydrates in an ounce, but since 11 of them come from fiber, an ounce of chia seeds clocks in at only 1 net carb, making them a low-carb, keto diet superfood.

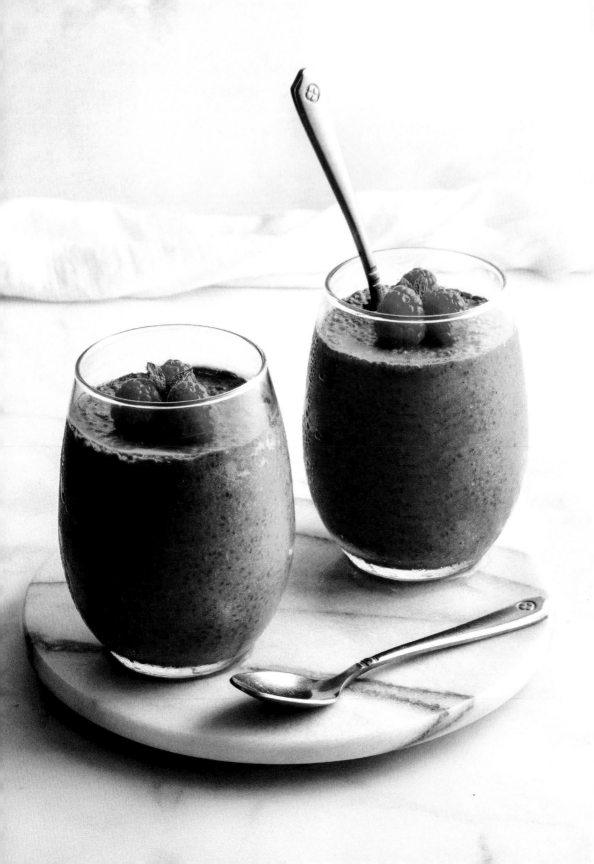

WHITE CHOCOLATE PECAN TRUFFLES

SERVES 2

These White Chocolate Pecan Truffles are easy to whip together, without turning the oven on, and incredibly delicious. If you don't have pecans, you can use walnuts in their place, but keep in mind that changes the carb count. An ounce of pecans has about 1 gram of net carbs, while the same amount of walnuts has 2 grams.

⅛ **cup pecans**

2 tablespoons cocoa butter

2 tablespoons coconut oil

⅛ **teaspoon vanilla extract**

3 drops liquid stevia

PER 1 TRUFFLE

Calories: 280
Fat: 30g
Protein: 1g
Sodium: 0mg
Fiber: 1g
Carbohydrates: 1g
Net Carbohydrates: 0g
Sugar: 0g

1 Chop pecans coarsely with a knife or process quickly in a food processor so they don't get too fine.

2 In a small saucepan over very low heat, add cocoa butter and coconut oil, stirring until completely melted, about 3 minutes.

3 Remove from heat and stir in pecans, vanilla extract, and stevia.

4 Pour into four silicone molds. Refrigerate 1 hour or until hardened.

5 Remove from molds. Serve immediately or store in refrigerator up to one week.

SWEET STEVIA

Stevia, which is a natural, no-calorie, no-carbohydrate sweetener, is approximately two hundred to three hundred times sweeter than regular sugar. Because it's so potent, you only need a tiny amount in any recipes that you make with it. If you want to use erythritol or a monk fruit sweetener blend in its place, you'll have to adjust the amounts accordingly, since it takes a little more of the other two to get the same sweetness factor as stevia.

PISTACHIO PUDDING

SERVES 2

After you try this homemade Pistachio Pudding, you will never look at the boxed stuff again. It's creamy and delicious, but the best part: It's good for you! Try to find natural pistachio flavoring instead of the sugar-free stuff that's full of artificial sweeteners.

5 ounces cream cheese, softened

3 tablespoons heavy whipping cream

4 drops liquid stevia

1 teaspoon natural pistachio flavoring

¼ cup crushed pistachios

1 In a medium bowl, beat cream cheese until light and fluffy, about 2 minutes. Add whipping cream and beat until smooth.

2 Beat in stevia and pistachio flavoring.

3 Stir in crushed pistachios.

4 Refrigerate until firm, about 45 minutes to 1 hour. Serve chilled.

PER SERVING

Calories: 412
Fat: 35g
Protein: 8g
Sodium: 267mg
Fiber: 2g
Carbohydrates: 8g
Net Carbohydrates: 6g
Sugar: 4g

POP SOME PISTACHIOS

Pistachios are high in fat, but they're also one of the nuts that are a little higher in carbs. One-fourth cup of crushed pistachios contains 5.25 grams of net carbohydrates. When including pistachios in your desserts or meals, make sure you're sticking to the portion sizes so that you're staying within your carbohydrate needs. If you don't have room for the extra carbs, you can use macadamia nuts instead.

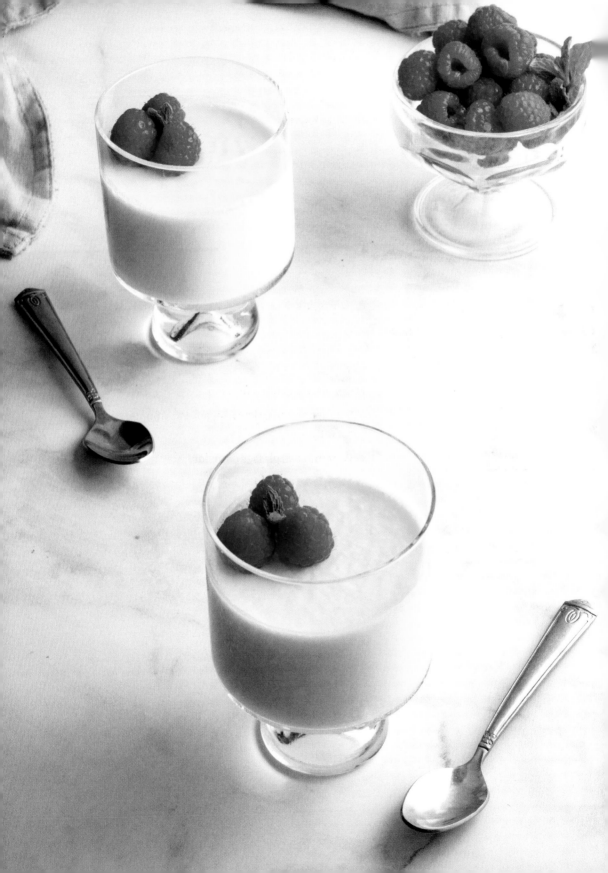

RASPBERRIES AND CREAM PANNA COTTA

SERVES 2

Raspberries are a low-carb fruit, providing only about 1.5 grams of net carbohydrates per ¼ cup. If you have some room in your carbohydrate allotment and want to add more berries to the top of your panna cotta, you can. You can also add some variation by using other low-carb berries like blueberries, blackberries, or even strawberries without changing the net carb count too much.

1 cup heavy whipping cream

1 teaspoon powdered unflavored grass-fed gelatin

1 tablespoon erythritol or granular Swerve

⅛ teaspoon raspberry flavor

6 fresh raspberries

PER SERVING

Calories: 417
Fat: 42g
Protein: 4g
Sodium: 46mg
Fiber: 0g
Carbohydrates: 10g
Net Carbohydrates: 7g
Sugar: 4g

1 Pour cream into a small saucepan, sprinkle gelatin on top, and let sit 5 minutes.

2 Add sweetener and raspberry flavor to saucepan. Place saucepan over low heat and whisk until ingredients are well blended, about 3 minutes.

3 Simmer over very low heat about 1 minute, stirring constantly.

4 Pour into two glasses or molds.

5 Refrigerate until set, at least 6 hours or overnight.

6 Top each dish with three raspberries and serve.

WHAT'S THE DEAL WITH GELATIN?

Gelatin, which is closely related to collagen, is a protein that's made by boiling the skin, tendons, ligaments, and bones of an animal (usually a cow or pig) to extract the nutrients in the marrow. The amino acids that you get from gelatin are hard to get from other foods. Including a high-quality, grass-fed source of the protein in your diet may help improve gut health and keep your hair, skin, and nails healthy. Although gelatin and collagen are similar, gelatin forms a gel when used in recipes, while collagen completely dissolves in water, so the two can't be used interchangeably in most cases.

MEYER LEMON PANNA COTTA

SERVES 2

Panna cotta is an easy keto-approved dessert that's a cinch to whip up when you want to have a quick dessert, but don't want to spend a lot of time fussing in the kitchen. It does require at least 6 hours of chill time, so make it the night before you want to eat it or in the morning so it's ready right after dinner.

1 cup full-fat coconut milk

1 teaspoon powdered unflavored grass-fed gelatin

1 tablespoon erythritol or granular Swerve

Zest of 1 medium Meyer lemon

1 tablespoon coconut oil

1 teaspoon fresh Meyer lemon juice

PER SERVING
Calories: 285
Fat: 29g
Protein: 3g
Sodium: 16mg
Fiber: 0g
Carbohydrates: 10g
Net Carbohydrates: 7g
Sugar: 0g

1 Pour coconut milk into a small saucepan, sprinkle gelatin on top, and let sit 5 minutes.

2 Add remaining ingredients to saucepan. Place saucepan over low heat and whisk until gelatin and zest are completely incorporated, about 3 minutes.

3 Simmer over very low heat about 1 minute, stirring constantly.

4 Pour into two glasses or molds.

5 Refrigerate until set, at least 6 hours or overnight.

6 Serve in glass or invert over a small plate after dipping glass into hot water a few seconds.

BUTTERSCOTCH CUSTARD

SERVES 2

If you're looking for a way to up your healthy fat intake in a sweet way, this Butterscotch Custard is it. It combines butter with heavy cream and egg yolk to make a decadent dessert that will make you both happy. If you use salted butter instead of unsalted, skip adding the extra salt.

1 tablespoon unsalted grass-fed butter

¼ cup erythritol or granular Swerve

½ cup heavy cream

1 large egg yolk

½ teaspoon vanilla extract

⅛ teaspoon sea salt

PER SERVING
Calories: 290
Fat: 29g
Protein: 3g
Sodium: 141mg
Fiber: 0g
Carbohydrates: 26g
Net Carbohydrates: 14g
Sugar: 2g

1 Preheat oven to 300°F.

2 Place two ramekins in a deep baking pan just large enough to hold them.

3 In a small saucepan over medium heat, melt butter and sweetener and cook until butter browns, about 5 minutes.

4 Very slowly add heavy cream, whisking constantly until completely blended with butter, about 5 minutes.

5 In a small bowl, whisk together remaining ingredients until egg yolk is foamy.

6 Slowly pour egg mixture into cream, whisking constantly to combine well.

7 Pour mixture through a fine strainer into ramekins using a spoon to help you.

8 Pour hot water into baking pan until it is halfway up the outside of ramekins. Bake until custard is set, about 35 minutes.

9 Remove from oven and let cool in baking pan about 4 hours. It can be stored in the refrigerator up to three days.

PUMPKIN DONUT HOLES

SERVES 2

These donut holes are the perfect bite-sized treat, especially around the holidays. Just make sure to use pure pumpkin purée instead of premade pumpkin pie filling, which is loaded with sugar and will up the carbohydrate count significantly.

½ cup almond flour

1 tablespoon granulated erythritol

⅛ teaspoon salt

¼ teaspoon baking soda

¼ tablespoon pumpkin pie seasoning

1 large egg

3 tablespoons canned pumpkin purée

1 tablespoon unsalted butter, melted

½ tablespoon cream cheese

¼ teaspoon vanilla extract

6 drops maple extract

1 Preheat oven to 325°F. Grease six wells of a mini muffin tin.

2 In a medium bowl, combine almond flour, erythritol, salt, baking soda, and pumpkin pie seasoning. Stir until combined.

3 In a small bowl, beat egg, pumpkin purée, melted butter, cream cheese, vanilla extract, and maple extract until smooth. Fold egg mixture into dry ingredients until just combined.

4 Drop by teaspoonfuls into each well of a mini muffin tin.

5 Bake 15 minutes or until a toothpick inserted in the center comes out clean. Store at room temperature.

PER SERVING
Calories: 275
Fat: 23g
Protein: 10g
Sodium: 351mg
Fiber: 4g
Carbohydrates: 15g
Net Carbohydrates: 8g
Sugar: 3g

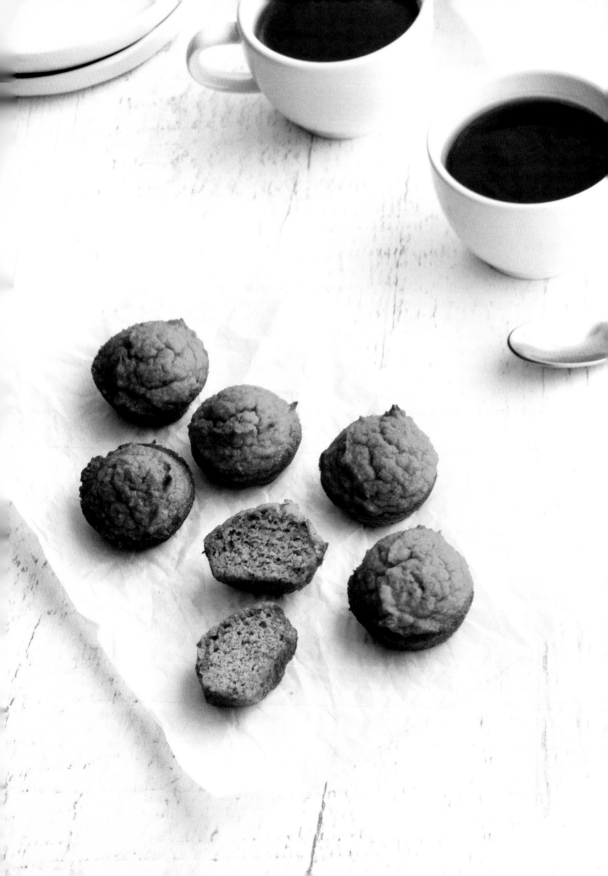

KEY LIME PIE SMOOTHIE

SERVES 2

This Key Lime Pie Smoothie gives you all the taste of a pie without all of the carbs. The heavy cream makes it rich and creamy while the gelatin holds everything together. You can throw everything in the blender after dinner and have a simple but delicious dessert for two in no time.

1½ cups heavy cream

2 tablespoons powdered unflavored grass-fed gelatin

2 teaspoons vanilla extract

3 tablespoons freshly squeezed key lime juice

2 teaspoons lime zest

⅛ teaspoon liquid stevia

12 ice cubes

1 Pour heavy cream and gelatin into a blender and blend to combine.

2 Add remaining ingredients except ice cubes and blend another minute until well mixed.

3 Place ice cubes into blender and process until smoothie thickens. Divide between two glasses and serve immediately.

PER SERVING
Calories: 657
Fat: 63g
Protein: 10g
Sodium: 78mg
Fiber: 0g
Carbohydrates: 8g
Net Carbohydrates: 8g
Sugar: 6g

US/METRIC CONVERSION CHART

VOLUME CONVERSIONS

US Volume Measure	Metric Equivalent
⅛ teaspoon	0.5 milliliter
¼ teaspoon	1 milliliter
½ teaspoon	2 milliliters
1 teaspoon	5 milliliters
½ tablespoon	7 milliliters
1 tablespoon (3 teaspoons)	15 milliliters
2 tablespoons (1 fluid ounce)	30 milliliters
¼ cup (4 tablespoons)	60 milliliters
⅓ cup	90 milliliters
½ cup (4 fluid ounces)	125 milliliters
⅔ cup	160 milliliters
¾ cup (6 fluid ounces)	180 milliliters
1 cup (16 tablespoons)	250 milliliters
1 pint (2 cups)	500 milliliters
1 quart (4 cups)	1 liter (about)

WEIGHT CONVERSIONS

US Weight Measure	Metric Equivalent
½ ounce	15 grams
1 ounce	30 grams
2 ounces	60 grams
3 ounces	85 grams
¼ pound (4 ounces)	115 grams
½ pound (8 ounces)	225 grams
¾ pound (12 ounces)	340 grams
1 pound (16 ounces)	454 grams

OVEN TEMPERATURE CONVERSIONS

Degrees Fahrenheit	Degrees Celsius
200 degrees F	95 degrees C
250 degrees F	120 degrees C
275 degrees F	135 degrees C
300 degrees F	150 degrees C
325 degrees F	160 degrees C
350 degrees F	180 degrees C
375 degrees F	190 degrees C
400 degrees F	205 degrees C
425 degrees F	220 degrees C
450 degrees F	230 degrees C

BAKING PAN SIZES

American	Metric
8 × 1½ inch round baking pan	20 × 4 cm cake tin
9 × 1½ inch round baking pan	23 × 3.5 cm cake tin
11 × 7 × 1½ inch baking pan	28 × 18 × 4 cm baking tin
13 × 9 × 2 inch baking pan	30 × 20 × 5 cm baking tin
2 quart rectangular baking pan	30 × 20 × 3 cm baking tin
15 × 10 × 2 inch baking pan	30 × 25 × 2 cm baking tin (Swiss roll tin)
9 inch pie plate	22 × 4 or 23 × 4 cm pie plate
7 or 8 inch springform pan	18 or 20 cm springform or loose bottom cake tin
9 × 5 × 3 inch loaf pan	23 × 13 × 7 cm or 2 lb narrow loaf or pâté tin
1½ quart casserole	1.5 liter casserole
2 quart casserole	2 liter casserole

INDEX